WHAT WENT
WRONG?

Pharma Tech Case Studies

Pharma Regulatory Investigations

P G SHROTRIYA

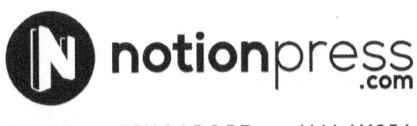

INDIA · SINGAPORE · MALAYSIA

Notion Press

Old No. 38, New No. 6
McNichols Road, Chetpet
Chennai - 600 031

First Published by Notion Press 2020
Copyright © P G Shrotriya 2020
All Rights Reserved.

ISBN

Paperback: 978-1-64850-658-1

Hardcase: 978-1-64899-759-4

Contents

Preamble

Academic institutions have been imparting knowledge of basic science and technology in pharmaceutical educational institutions in India since 1932. It started as a need-based education. Over the years, drugs and the pharmaceutical industry have made phenomenal progress achieving international recognition. In 2018, the industry achieved a turnover of about Rs.1268 billion (US $ 18.12 billion) (McKinsey). It's expected to reach about Rs 2933Billion (US $ 41.9 Bill.) by FY20. Phenomenal progress! It not only meets the country's requirements but exports world over, including the US, where it exports about 40% of their requirements of API and generic drug products. It has achieved the highest number of US FDA approved facilities in India, next to the US! It is recognised as World Pharmacy.

Thanks to academia in the country that provided human resources to the industry. Government policies also made a significant contribution to these achievements. The industry has achieved global recognition through their endeavour to meet international standards with arduous efforts. Yet, there is a need to support the industry by academia, with updated knowledge and training of young graduates, postgraduates and doctorates with a globally accepted standard of subjects, including ethics and ethical values.

Essentially, knowledge and training imparted to students remain within the theoretical and practical exposure of teachers in industrial working. There is a need to impart a problem-solving capability/approach in academic institutions. Lack of this is a serious issue the industry is facing.

The president of India expressed his concern, in one of his convocation addresses, over the quality of higher education in the country. McKinsey has observed that fresh graduates and postgraduates lack applicative aspect in a real work situation.

Students take a few months to settle and understand working requirements in the industry since they are trained in theoretical learning. Practical exposure to working in the industry is lacking, and academia is unable to provide the same due to lack of insight.

Transfer of knowledge depends on the capability of an individual teacher, which limits the integrated multidisciplinary approach. Due to lake of integrated knowledge, new entrants to the industry struggle to learn it in a hard way.

The industry is looking at global business (once having reached turnover of about Rs.50 Cr about US $ 7 Million business), and mere theoretical training is inadequate to understand and meet current global regulatory compliance. Any issue in the industry of market/consumer complaint has to be understood comprehensively, and the solution has to be of scientific and technical relevance. The applicative multidisciplinary approach suggesting corrective action and preventive action (CAPA) is desirable to ensure that a similar situation is averted in the future.

Practical training in the industry should be compulsory for at least six months. It must be looked at as an opportunity to understand the working with science and technology and not a cut-paste/quick-fix approach. Learning comes only on working with once own hands and not with a supervisory approach. Real learning comes from working with operators/technician and gaining knowledge of tricks of the trade. The inquisitive approach will impart self-learning with confidence.

The objective of this book is to provide multidisciplinary approaches/guidelines for problem-solving capability. These case studies are based on the actual situation faced and successfully resolved with a back-up of science and technology convincing international regulators/complainants, leading to the closing of complaints.

Abbreviations

AR   :   Analytical Report
BMR   :   Batch Manufacturing Record
BPR   :   Batch Packaging Record
CAPA   :   Corrective Action and Preventive Action
COA   :   Certificate of Analysis
DI   :   Data Integrity
HPH   :   High Pressure Homogeniser
IPQC   :   In-Process Quality Control
IPC   :   In-Process Control
NS   :   Nano Sizer
PIL   :   Patient Information Leaflet
QA   :   Quality Assurance
QC   :   Quality Control
QP   :   Qualified Person
RC   :   Radius of Curvature
Temp   :   Temperature
WA   :   Water Activity

Acknowledgements

Case studies presented in this book are out of my industrial experience over the last four decades in India and overseas. Irrespective of organisation, investigation to arrive at assignable reason is a mammoth exercise and require help and support from various departments within the organisation and overseas customers/and regulatory agencies. It requires a multifaceted and applicative approach. It involves an out-of-the-box approach in resolving issues faced within the country/ overseas. All possible alternatives have to be explored to find an assignable reason for the issue. It requires centralised control approach with time-bound thinking to ensure resolution within the time frame committed to regulators/customers.

Many scientific and technical brains were involved, some of them with a dedicated approach with marathon discussions, some as doers not leaving any facet of investigations. Lead players of the investigations deserve to be acknowledged for their contribution in resolving the issues.

Contribution of few lead participants, from different organisations, who supported me in investigations and arriving at assignable scientific reason acceptable to the customer/organisation/regulators – Mr S. Parthsarthy, Mr M. Hemadri, Mr A. Shah, Mr H.H. Pandit, Mr Hitesh Bhatt, Mr A. Desai, Mr S. Rami, Mr Kirti Maheshwari, Mr R. Tuljapurkar, Mr A. Joshi, Mr D Joshi, Mr S Roy, Mr S Makoday, Mr A Mukhariya and Mr J.Raval – are gratefully acknowledged. I appreciate, with thanks, the contribution and support of other technical and non-technical participants.

Encouragement from Prof Ram Gaud to write this book is thankfully acknowledged.

I acknowledge, with thanks, the support of Smita Shrotriya, Kunal Shrotriya, Richa Shrotriya and Kinjal Desai, throughout this effort.

Foreword

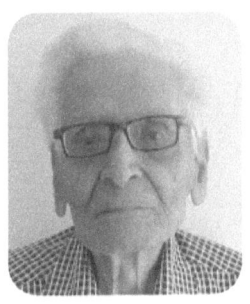

S. N. Sharma

Professor Emeritus,
Hamdard University, New Delhi

The father of Dr. P G Shrotriya started pharmacy (pharmacy – Dispensing Chemists and Druggists shop) in 1946. This was the beginning of his interest in pharmacy right from his childhood. With this background, when he grew, he decided to join a pharmacy course and did his B.Pharm. M.Pharm. and PhD from Saugor University. His love for teaching first took him to an academic institution.

However, he was more inclined to use his knowledge in the industry, which took him to pharmaceutical industries – Tamil Nadu Dadha Pharmaceutical Ltd, Madras (now Chennai), followed by Warner Hindustan, Hyderabad, Helios Pharmaceuticals, Ahmedabad, M. J. Pharmaceuticals (technical tie-up with Eli Lilly – USA), Baroda, Ranbaxy Laboratories, Dewas, Intas Pharmaceuticals, Ahmedabad, M.J. Biopharm, New Mumbai and Cadila Pharmaceuticals, Ahmedabad. He was exposed to every facet of the pharmaceutical industry for 40 years.

Having gained significant all-round experience, he started the Elite Consultancy Services (Pharmaceutical Consultancy Services) as CEO. He worked for a number of organisations on techno-commercial projects, including greenfield projects in India and overseas. He worked for WHO as a global resource person and contributed to several international standards, acknowledged in a number of the WHO's technical reports.

Indian pharmaceutical industries essentially work i) for exports only, ii) for the Indian market only and iii) Indian and export markets. Each one of them requires compliance with the respective regulatory requirements.

Having worked in several Pharma industries, he had opportunities to face a number of National and International Regulatory Agencies, to mention some of them – US, UK, EU, WHO and Australia, etc. He faced the first inspection of the US FDA and UK MCA (Now MHRA) in India and obtained their approvals and exported pharmaceutical products to them. This required compliance to international GMP and GLP requirements for R&D, warehouse, QC, QA, manufacturing, engineering services, packaging, supply chain, including distribution, recalls, exports and regulatory covering all dosage forms such as solid orals, oral liquids, semisolids, injectable – liquids, unit lyophilised and biotech products beside environmental controls.

I am reminded of my friend, Mr. Shivanand K. Kattishettar, then Drugs Controller, Karnataka State. I was with him in his office when he received a telephone call from then Drugs Controller of India asking him to withdraw a batch of Heparin injections, which exceeded its label claim of the drug, which could be disastrous for any patient. He swiftly approached regulators in different parts of Karnataka to stop sell and withdrew the batch. This revealed the swift and tough action to be taken by the regulator in public interest.

He was exposed to every facet of the pharmaceutical industry in India and overseas; Dr Shrotriya also shared his experience with pharmacy graduates, postgraduates, PhD students and teachers of several universities, besides NMIMS University, Nirma University and Regulatory Agencies in India and overseas.

He conducted a number of continuing education training for faculty members of several universities in India and delivered lectures to an international audience, to mention a few: i) Nanjing, China – "Pharma Tech Case Studies, What Went Wrong?" ii) Boston, USA – "Pharma Tech Case Studies, What Went Wrong? – Regulatory Investigation" iii) Osaka, Japan – "Innovations in Pharmaceutical Sciences – Help of Nature, Regenerative Medicines and Nanotechnology" iv) Key Note Address at 8th Pharma Middle East Congress, Dubai, UAE v) International Society For Pharmaceutical Engineering (ISPE Conference), Bologna (Italy) vi) Dhaka (Bangladesh) vii) Kathmandu (Nepal) viii) Damascus (Syria) ix) Addis Ababa (Ethiopia), etc. He shared his professional experience in innovations and regulatory compliance.

Considering his vast industrial experience, integrating multidisciplinary approach, case studies in this book will benefit students, academia, industry, professionals, regulatory agencies and hospitals providing guidelines in finding the solution to their issues.

I congratulate Dr P G Shrotriya for his initiative in writing his experience, in this book – *What Went Wrong? Pharma Tech Case Studies*

New Delhi, India.

S. N. Sharma

Professor Emeritus,
Hamdard University, New Delhi

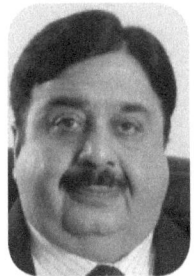

 PHARMACY COUNCIL OF INDIA

(Constituted under the Pharmacy Act 1948)

Prof. B. Suresh M.Pharm., Ph.D., D.Sc.
President

Combined Councils' Building
Kotla Road, Aiwan-E- Ghalib Marg
P.B. No. 7020, New Delhi-110 002
Phone: 011 23239184, 23231348. Fax: 011 23239184

Vice-Chancellor, JSS University
Sri Shivarathreeshwara Nagar, Mysuru-570 015
Phone: 0821 2548391 Fax: 0821 2548394
sureshbhojiraj@gmail.com
sureshjssuni@hotmail.com
www.jssuni.edu.in

FOREWORD

Drugs and Pharmaceutical Industry in India has achieved enviable position in production and supply of generic drugs and pharmaceuticals of international standards to Indian population and several other countries including developed nations.

For every organisation, despite adhering to regulatory norms, do come across a situation / instances, when it receives (market) complaint either from customer or regulatory agency, or observations made by an individual while working, which calls for attention to avoid serious issue in future. This is where the book *What* Went Wrong? authored by Dr P G Shrotriya attempts to present some of the case studies, their investigations and corrective action taken with an objective to share his experience with professionals and faculty and students. Documentation is the area which has attracted wrath (attention) of regulators – for inadequacy in information / no information / unacceptable or doubtful results. Systematic investigation is required for any complaint to arrive at satisfactory response to the complainant. Gross inadequacy in response has been observed with casual / half-hearted attempt without ascertaining the reason! Many a time response to a complaint is looked at as a ritual for compliance!

For organisation, satisfaction of regulator or a complainant is a business process for a progressive industry. Remember, pharma industry caters the requirements of millions of ailing population where, there is no seconds, and no one can take a chance.

As a Pharmacy professional, my experience has taught me how valuable a handbook like this is for students and readers. In this perspective, I sincerely appreciate the efforts and farsightedness of the author. Objective of this book is to provide multidisciplinary approach / guidelines for problem solving capability. These case studies are based on actual situation faced and successfully resolved with back-up of science and technology convincing international regulators leading to closing of complaints.

I am sure that this book will be valued by its readers not merely as a theoretically-oriented venture, but also as a hands-on-guide to tackle problems pertaining thereof. I congratulate and express my best wishes to the authors for bringing out this publication.

Dr B Suresh
President

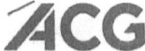

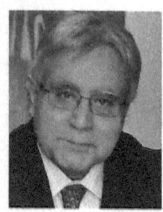

AJIT SINGH

CHAIRMAN – ACG (Formerly Associated Capsules Group)

Foreword

India is perhaps the only Country in the world where a majority of students of pharmacy join the Pharmaceutical Industry. In almost all other Countries, pharmacy graduates enter retail pharmacy, community pharmacy, hospital pharmacy and the like.

With this knowledgeable and unique resource, India has been able to lead the world in the production and export of generic pharma formulations. India is able to make vast quantities of medicines, of international standard quality in the world in a most effective manner.

Other Countries have not been able to match India's leadership. This has brought recognition for the Country and is a valuable source of export earnings.

Dr. Shrotriya has been an important and early player in India's journey, both in preparing young pharmacists and then playing a key role in Industry as well. Interestingly, Dr. Shrotriya is one of the few who have successfully moved from Academia to Industry. He spent a decade and a half in teaching and academic research. He was a Teacher, Adjunct Professor, Director – Pharmaceutical Research and Visiting Faculty at a number of Colleges of Pharmacy in Maharashtra, Gujarat and other states in India.

Showing considerable flexibility and initiative Dr. Shrotriya then moved on to a new career in Industry. For several decades he held senior positions in global and domestic pharmaceutical companies. Moving from Senior Manager to General Manager to Senior Vice-President to whole time Director. He has finally started his own pharmaceutical consultancy firm, imparting International Regulatory Compliance advice, as well as GMP, GEP, and GCP auditing for leading Indian and Western pharma companies.

In this book readers will find many Pharma case studies covering what went wrong? and the correctives.

His career has been an example for those in academia, who would like to acquire courage and initiative to step out into the hustle and bustle of Industry.

Regd. Office :
1001, Dalamal House, Nariman Point, Mumbai - 400 021, India.
Phone : +91 22 2287 2557-2559

ACG

I came in contact with Dr. Shrotriya when he was whole-time Director of M J Pharma (Gujarat). He joined comprehensive facility of M J Pharma (near Baroda) in collaboration with Eli Lilly of the USA. It involved Transfer of Technology in the late 1980's for very sensitive lyophilized injectable and human insulin product lines from an advanced Country to a relatively lesser developed district in India. It was a pioneering effort at its time and, demonstrated it could be done.

As part of this process Dr. Shrotriya piloted M J Pharma to become the first to obtain US FDA, MHRA (then MCA) approvals for the plant in India, and exported products to US and UK.

Even while involved in Industry, Dr. Shrotriya found time to serve on the Indian Pharmacopoeia Commission – chairing their Parental Committee.

He also worked as a WHO Global resource person for Drugs and Pharmaceuticals and was acknowledged in several WHO Technical Reports. As a member of the Committee of the National Formulary of India, he contributed an Appendix on Disposal of unused and expired Pharmaceutical products.

This showed an admirable prescience of future health concerns. The importance of waste disposal has now become a major pre-occupation of Industry and the Regulatory Authorities, as is also of public concern.

In addition to his other duties Dr. Shrotriya continued his learning and academic pursuits. He delivered lectures to Professional Bodies, Regulatory Authorities and Universities in several Countries, and continued as a PhD examiner and Selection Committee Member for several institutions.

Organizing three Pharmaceutical Congress Dr. Shrotriya demonstrated rare organizational capabilities in leading and motivating a Committee of top Industry professionals, Company heads and Regulators, working Pro-bono, with some of them senior to him.

I was in close contact with Dr. Shrotriya when we were on the Founding Committee of the International Society of Pharmaceutical Engineering, (ISPE) India, an affiliate of the Global body. He displayed high energy, vast experience, Industry insight and considerable analytical skills. The ISPE India was recognized as the best world-wide affiliate in its second year.

In his long and illustrious career Dr.Shrotriya has played an integral role in the development of the Pharma Industry and Academia, and has interacted with innumerable global Regulatory Authorities.
For all the above reasons, among others, I look forward to the publication of his book, with its practical contents and case studies. We can all benefit from Dr. Shrotriya's experience and wisdom.

In fact, I plan to acquire many copies of his book to be sent to colleagues in Industry, Academia and Regulatory Bodies around the World.

Ajit Singh – Chairman
ACG- (Formerly Associated Capsules Group)

Introduction

The Drugs and Pharmaceutical Industry in India has achieved an enviable position in the production and supply of generic drugs and pharmaceuticals of international standards to the Indian population and several other countries, including developed nations, e.g., it caters about 40% requirements of generic drugs and pharmaceuticals to the US. This is realised due to the positive contribution of the policy of the Government of India. Academia has also contributed significantly in this process, providing human resources to the industry.

For every organisation, despite adhering to regulatory norms, does come across a situation/instance when it receives (market) complaint either from a customer or a regulatory agency or observations made by an individual while working, which calls for attention to avoid more serious issues in the future. The author has attempted to present some of the case studies, their investigations and the corrective actions taken with an objective to share his experience with professionals, teachers, students, investigators and regulators as a part of continuing education programme – a lifelong learning process.

Remember, when the world's worst possible disaster happens, it'll seldom be due to the failure of machinery or a system. Behind such instances is the human factor – people are responsible. It could be due to overlooking risk or consequences, keeping aside dictates of science and technology or quick-fix approach. Analysis reveals assignable reason for the event and learning the lesson the hard way, e.g., the Bhopal Disaster of 2nd Dec 1984 in India.

For the organisation, it could be very costly in terms of image, due to adverse publicity and impression created on regulators, patients and the public at large. With the growth of an organisation, there is a greater need to mechanise quality assurance requirements to avoid/ minimise man-made/overlooked errors. This assures shift to machine dependence from man – where human behaviour/mood frequency impact significantly on quality assurance.

Documentation is the area that has attracted wrath (attention) of regulators – for the inadequacy of information/no information/unacceptable or doubtful results/questionable data integrity. A systematic investigation is required for any complaint to arrive at a satisfactory response to the complainant. Gross inadequacy, in response, has been observed with casual/ half-hearted attempt without ascertaining the reason! Many a time, the response to a complaint is looked at as a ritual for compliance!

There is a gross mismatch even in the industry. Pharmacists in the industry do not have adequate knowledge of pharmaceutical machinery, and engineers lack knowledge of drugs and pharmaceuticals. Pharmacists shy away from handling machinery! During inspections, international regulators ask supervisors to demonstrate the working of the machinery, and they blink since they never operated it! This creates embarrassing situations for them. The fact is in academic institutions, the course content of pharmaceutical engineering does require the inclusion of important aspects of pharmaceutical machinery or interpretation of machine/tools drawing as the syllabus does not cover! Teachers and students must encourage a multidisciplinary approach in their understanding of subjects and practice to be successful in an industry working environment.

Microbiology is another area that needs to be strengthened. Present knowledge does not reflect the requirements of Pharmacopoeia. Many consider it is not required due to lack of education/exposure to appreciate its importance.

Many students shy away from chemistry due to lack of interest/poor knowledge! Without a back-up of chemistry, it is difficult to resolve issues – be it in R&D, bulk drug, manufacturing, QC, packaging or analytical development or reactivity of drugs and excipients with machine/tooling parts/primary packing material in drugs and pharmaceutical industry.

A casual approach, in response to observations of a regulator, leads to questionable data integrity! The number of warning letters issued to industries by international regulators on data integrity indicates the habitual approach of and acceptance of the same by supervisor(s) is alarming! This leads to a lack of confidence/trust by the regulator(s) in people working in the organisation. Remember, doubt in capability at an international level leads to distrust on even research publications from the country, leading to a crisis of confidence.

During one of the interactions with the international regulator, he raised a query on whether academia had a role/control in such an event, leading to the adoption of the wrong practices by youngsters in the industry? This is a reflection of human behaviour. Can we/how do we control?

This has shaken up the confidence of regulators and industry. It needs serious thinking both by academia and supervisors controlling activities in the industry.

For academia and organisation, the only way out is continuous training and the development of people with practical orientation ensuring regulatory compliance, resisting wrong practices/short cuts. Strict implementation of ethical practices as a part of academic training and business development is desirable.

This will depend on how do we strengthen the subject – Regulatory in academia? Change in approach to the subject is desirable. Maybe the involvement of the regulatory agency having working experience in industry or an experienced person from industry and the training of teachers for applied regulatory could help! An integrated approach of the subject regulatory with every other subject in academia may help in bringing home importance and application of regulatory in a work situation meeting compliance, which is the industry's requirement. This will go a long way in building confidence in academia, international and national regulators with image building of the industry and eventually that of the country.

For the organisation, the satisfaction of a regulator or a complainant is a business process for a progressive industry. Remember, the Pharma industry caters the requirements of millions of ailing population where there are no seconds, and no one can take a chance. Only shop floor training is inadequate without back-up support of science, technology and ethics.

It is mandatory to have an institutional ethics committee. People associated with the ethics committee should be exposed to Regulatory requirements. They must have adequate knowledge of the subject/exposed to the needs for any ethical scientific investigations. Else, it remains as an eyewash/ritual. Pharmaceutical investigations are quite complex, and those who had no exposure cannot appreciate/insist on requirements.

Academia has been meeting requirements of industry and regulators. However, they need to stretch extra to meet national and international regulatory requirements. Maybe the Pharmacy Council of India could play a role in training and development of teachers involving a knowledgeable person(s) from the industry as a partner for the ultimate benefit of future professionals, industry and the country!

Documentation of Complaint and Investigation

Access to documents for investigation is restricted to an authorised person in QA and controlled with records of persons who had access.

Each complaint received from regulatory agency/ customer has to be documented with details, as suggested in the following format including investigations carried out and CAPA derived, including the acceptance of the investigation by the regulatory agency/customer form a part of the record.

Format for the Regulatory/Market Complaint and Investigation Report

1. Complaint No.: Date

2. Originated from place/Country:

3. Name and detail address of the complainant/ regulatory agency:

4. Details of the product under complaint:

   Name of the product, strength, packing, Batch/ Lot No., manufacturing and expiry date, address of manufacturer and packer, details of primary, secondary and tertiary packing, whether repacked, the origin of complaint place – country/level of primary and secondary transportation subjected to, no. of loading – unloading undertaken, temp and RH on arrival, data logger (returned by the customer on receipt of the consignment) information on transit temp and RH and time duration in total transit-transportation.

5. Details/Description of Complaint:

6. Injury/damage/death of patient(s):

7. Information in detail received from Regulatory Agency/Complainant:

8. Protocol and investigation carried out (Sequence of Investigation):

9. Assignable reason for the complaint:

10. Corrective Action Preventive Action (CAPA) emerged:

11. Communication to Regulatory Agency/Complainant:

12. Acceptance response from the Regulatory Agency/Complainant:

13. Additional information required, if any:

14. Closing of the Complaint:

Investigator Name: Approved By Name:

Position: Position:

Date and Place: Date and Place:

CASE Study 1

Ethambutol Tablets BP

Ethambutol Tablets BP, 500 mg, was regularly manufactured and exported to a number of countries without any complaint. Overseas customer (regulatory agency) reported, after one year of receipt of the consignment, that the product had a typical odour! The product had a leftover life of one of the two years of shelf life (expiry date).

Product Pack Profile: Ethambutol Tablets BP 500 mg – 500 tablets were packed in a 300 gauge low-density polyethylene bag and sealed and labelled. This, in turn, packed a tin container, having aluminium tagger with appropriate labelling on the container. Twelve such containers were packed in a 5 Ply, 150 GSM corrugated craft paper each, for box and partitions. The box was carry strapped with polypropylene strap. Two thousand such containers were exported to an overseas customer in Geneva.

The complaint was acknowledged, indicating that we would revert with the assignable reason and the investigation report in four to six weeks.

Investigations

1. Initially, the complaint was taken casually and responded to the customer that we have examined our manufacturing and QC records and no abnormality observed (typical QA response to the market complaint)!

2. Not satisfied with the response, the Regulator wrote to the Chairman of the Co., who in turn spoke and referred to the Executive Director.

3. The Regulator was told that we would come back with the investigation report in about 40 day time and requested for a sample from the batch under question for our investigation.

Protocol for the Investigation and Action Taken

1. Manufacturing and packaging batch records of the product, QC reports of all raw materials – API, excipients, packaging materials, purified water were examined, leading to no clue to the issue.

2. Environmental control records of the dispensing, manufacturing, packaging area, personnel record of individual involved in dispensing, manufacturing and packaging activities verified that they were not suffering from any disease; no abnormality was observed. Retention samples of API, excipients, product/packs were checked and reanalysed including microbiology; no abnormality was observed, including three batches, each before and after the batch in question.

3. After the complaint samples container received from the overseas customer, retention samples of previous five batches (to complaint) of finished products, including corresponding batches of API were examined for odour referred in the complaint. All the batches of the finished products and API revealed a similar odour to that of complaint sample!

4. All API and finished product samples were re-examined for total analysis as per BP, including microbiology. All samples complied with the BP specification.

5. Critical examination of API – Ethambutol BP specification revealed Related Substance Test for N – Butanol with a limit of 0.1%. Reference standard of this was examined for odour. It revealed an identical odour to that of the complaint sample and in retention samples of other batches of finished products!

6. Complaint samples along with that of retention samples of the complaint batch and other batches of finished products were tested again for Related Substance – N – Butanol and found complying with the BP test limit of 0.1% (found 0.04 to 0.05%)! Current BP specification is not more than 1.0%.

7. The odour and taste of API and finished products do not form a part of the specification in any Pharmacopoeia for obvious reason. However, such market complaint samples, QC and QA had undertaken the same to arrive at the assignable reason for the complaint.

8. A detailed report of the entire investigation was shared with the overseas Regulator, who agreed with the entire investigation and appreciated the efforts taken by the organisation. They admitted that it was also learning for them.

9. Regulator closed the complaint and agreed to request of the organisation to release use of the product which was quarantined.

CAPA

i. PIL of the product was amended to include "Product has a characteristic odour of the drug". COA of the product was amended to include odour.

ii. QC, QA chemists and supervisors were trained for the investigation.

CASE Study 2

Grievance of Industry Representative

<hr>

It was the International Conference organised by the International Society for Pharmaceutical Engineering (ISPE) at Bologna, Italy. This was the well-coordinated efforts of the Pharma industry, Pharma machinery manufacturers and academia. I was invited as a speaker. In the question-answer session, one of the Pharma industry representatives had a question, which was put up to me.

QUESTION: Sir, I am from a pharmaceutical industry that manufactures different generic tablet products. The EU Inspector visits us for GMP inspection. Ours is a small manufacturing and marketing company, and we have to meet the marketing requirements of different products. Marketing demands vary in size for products. We have standardised a validated batch size for different products. However, depending on market requirements, we do require to alter batch sizes since we cannot afford to keep the leftover inventory for an indefinite period in an unpacked condition. Hence, we make a batch size to meet marketing requirements, which involves the use of different tablet compression machines – 16 Station / 27 Station/45 Station rotary tablet compression machine. We did the process validation on 16 station tableting machines when we introduced the product. The EU inspectors insisted that we carry out process validation when we change the tableting machine. I have explained that our marketing requirements vary from time to time and management expects to accommodate marketing requirements. Please explain to me, is it rational on the part of EU Inspector to expect process validation when we change the tableting machine from 16 to 27 to 45 station for a product?

RESPONSE: This is a typical issue the Pharma industry faces during the stabilisation stage, and you need to satisfy GMP regulatory requirements. There is a science, technology and pharmaceutical engineering considerations for this.

When you carried out process validation for 16 station tableting machine, you must have considered particle size of API and that of all excipients, granule size of dried granules. Compacting force on punches will be different on 16/27/45 station tableting machine. Besides this, remember that dual time will be variable on 16/27/45 station. Hence, you need to alter compacting force to meet quality standards of physical and dissolution requirements of your tablet product. Do include frequency distribution of your lubricated granules since micromeritics play a very important role in the compressional behaviour of granules.

I suggest you include the particle size of API, excipients and frequency distribution of your granules as a part of your initial validation. Include details of frequency distribution data of granules of at least five batches on each tableting machine 16/27/45 station along with data of physical parameters and that of dissolution. Include this data as a part of process validation studies over a period of time. I am sure you will have a one-time effort as a solution to satisfy any regulator. I also suggest that include tablet tooling drawing as a part of validation data. This will facilitate your regulatory compliance also to satisfy and meet their requirements. Thereby, you will also establish yourself and organisation as science and technology-based. This will go a long way in confidence-building in regulators.

RESPONSE OF THE PERSON: I am satisfied and will do what you suggested. Thanks for your solution to the issue.

CASE Study 3

Ibuprofen Tablets BP

◈ ·································· ◈

(Product for Export – In-house issue)

The organisation was regularly supplying Ibuprofen Tablets BP to several countries as per their requirements. A batch under manufacturing suddenly encountered a blue spot on the biconvex surface of core tablets during initial compression trial. Attempts were made to resolve the issue, but it could not be solved.

Investigations:

The matter was brought to the notice of the supervisor and then to the departmental head. QC and QA were informed, and production was stopped, pending investigation and resolution of the issue.

The following course of the investigation was initiated:

1. Checking of bulk granules for bluish impurity encountered – bluish impurity was not observed in the bulk granules.

2. QC reports of all raw materials, including API used in the batch, were examined. QC reports of none of the materials revealed any clue!

3. The tableting machine was dismantled – hopper, chute, feed frame, upper and lower punches and dies were removed. All the parts were cleaned, including the turret, and refixed by the operator.

4. On restarting the machine, there were no blue spots. However, after running it for about 15 minutes, it reappeared on the upper surface!

5. Feed frame and upper punches were removed and cleaned.

6. The inner surface of the feed frame was observed with some sticky material with bluish colour!

7. The feed frame was thoroughly cleaned and refixed with a feeler gauge to ensure that distance between turret and feed frame was appropriately adjusted.

8. Compression was restarted, and the issue appeared to have been resolved.

9. The supervisor was entrusted with the responsibility to remain there until the batch was completed.

10. QA was entrusted to assure that no more blue spots were observed.

11. Earlier compressed tablets with blue spots were discarded.

Assignable Reason:

1. All raw materials, including API – Ibuprofen specification, were examined.

2. Chemical structure of Ibuprofen revealed that it has a phenyl propionic acid present in the structure of the NSAID. Further, it revealed that it has a melting point of 75-78°C.

3. The material of construction of the feed frame was made of phosphor-bronze.

4. A further in-depth study revealed that bronze contains a significant amount of copper in its composition.

5. Green spots were removed from tablets and underneath feed frame and analysed. It was found to contain Ibuprofen and traces of copper.

6. The shoe of the feed frame was found warm! Due to friction.

7. Improper adjustment – tightening of the feed frame shoe resulted into friction between the shoe and rotating turret, resulting in the warming of the shoe outlet, which in turn softened (acidic) Ibuprofen (m.p.75-78°C) and reacted with the copper of the bronze-Feed frame. The reaction between copper and Ibuprofen forming copper salt – bluish-green colour.

   Learning – Use of proper feeler gauge was made compulsory in adjusting space between shoe and turret. R&D chemists, operators, supervisors, engineers and QA and QC persons were trained to understand the importance of chemical nature, structure and activity/reactivity of drugs. Use of feeler gauge, pharmaceutical engineering – the role of machine parts and understanding of their material of construction and their likely reactivity was explained.

CAPA

i.   Change control was made for the use of the feeler gauge.

ii. SOP was made for the use of feeler gauge for space adjustment.

iii. Details of the issue, the investigation carried out, and resolution of the issue was included in the batch record.

iv. All batch manufacturing records (BMR) of different products were amended to include use of appropriate feeler gauge and recording of the same in respective BMR.

v.   R&D pharmacists, operators, supervisors, engineers, QA and QC persons were trained for the use of feeler gauge. They were also trained for understanding chemical nature, structure-activity/reactivity of drugs, pharmaceutical engineering – the role of machine parts, their material of construction and their likely reactivity.

vi. Master BMRs were amended, and International regulators were informed, and it was discussed with them during their subsequent inspection visit.

CASE Study 4

Environmental Control

The organisation was approved by MCA (now MHRA) for general products solid dosage forms, oral liquid, semisolid preparations and injectable facilities, including biotech liquid injectable and unit lyophilised cephalosporin injectable.

Preventive maintenance by engineering services was scheduled for the plant, once in a year during a lean period of activity. This also covered all utilities, including HVAC systems. All individual HVAC systems were checked for ΔP (pressure differential), and coarse filters were cleaned. Based on ΔP, in the biotech liquid filling station, HEPA filters were replaced. On completion of preventive maintenance work, the plant was scheduled to undertake working after particle count, adjusting ΔP and Temperature followed by media fill.

The biotech liquid injectable area was under recommissioning for starting a media fill. The area was sanitised for the environmental microbial count. Initially, viable counts were high and found the same even after repeated trials!

Investigation

The area was resenitised but did not comply with environmental microbiology standard! The matter was discussed with the technical group of the business partner – Multinational Company based in the US, with whom the organisation had a tie-up for supplies of finished products in Europe. The technical group in the US was provided with all the preventive maintenance work details. They assured to discuss the issue at their end and revert. The group reverted with a suggestion to take up the matter with a professor of microbiology in the university who was conducting training for them in the US.

Two-three suggestions discussed, during the tripartite telephonic meeting with the US group and the professor, tried but did not resolve the issue. The prof. had a look at the environmental microbiology data sent to her. Sanitiser was changed to another one, previously used in routine cyclic change, which did not resolve the issue. The professor suggested sanitising the area using routine sanitiser for the environment after checking RH in the area and adjusting it to 70% ± 5% and temp control of 22-25°C. Air sampling was done. The results indicated effective compliance with a much lower value than the earlier data! Environmental microbiology study was repeated. Repeat study data were found very satisfactory, in line with the earlier routine results. The US professor and representatives of the multinational Pharma Company were acknowledged with thanks for their help. They were informed of the data of both the studies.

Assignable Reason

The professor explained that for effective sanitisation, you needed to maintain RH 70% ± 5% beside temp control of 22°C-25°C. You require 70% RH to permeate the sanitising agent inside microbial cells.

CAPA

i. SOP was amended for the liquid injectable area to indicate temp and RH before sanitisation with change control.

ii. All master documents and BMRs were amended to include temp and RH data before aerial sanitisation in the liquid injectable area.

iii. Supervisors of production, QC, QA, engineers and operators were trained for basic microbiology with the rationale of maintaining temp and RH data record before undertaking environmental microbiology sampling.

iv. Regulatory agency was informed of the change control and amendment in the SOP with data.

CASE Study 5

Fluoxetine Capsules BP

❖ ·· ❖

The organisation was exporting the drug product to customers in the UK. However, in one of the supplies to a customer, the QP of the testing laboratory in the UK reported, through a business partner, that the batch complied with all the tests except for the weight of the content of capsule!

QP was acknowledged receipt of the complaint, indicating that we would revert with the assignable reason and the investigation report in four to six weeks.

Pack Profile

The Fluoxetine Capsules BP, 20 mg – ten capsules were packed in a blister pack of 0.025mm thick lacquered aluminium foil/0.25mm thick PVC. Each blister was packed in a printed carton with a patient information leaflet (PIL). Twenty such packs were packed in a corrugated box of 3ply 150 GSM craft paper. The box was sealed with adhesive tape. The product was exported along with a data logger through a container to the UK by sea.

Investigation

On receipt of the product complaint, the customer was requested to provide one of the packs of the unopened corrugated box (20 blister packs) along with the data logger, which was sent with the consignment for temp/RH monitoring in transit.

Retention samples of the batch product were examined by QA/QC. The batch manufacturing record (BMR) along with batch packaging record (BPR) were scrutinised for any discrepancy. QC records of all raw materials, including API used in the batch, were examined, awaiting the arrival of the shipper pack from the UK.

The customer was informed that we received the samples and investigating the matter and will revert in six weeks.

On receipt of complaint sample pack shipper, samples were analysed along with that of the retention samples as per BP specification. It complied with all the tests as per BP, except the weight of the content of capsules in case of complaint samples, which was found higher than the one reported in the QC report sent to the customer!

Retention samples of all raw materials, including API used in the batch, were reanalysed. BMR was examined in totality. Starch (dried) was used in the batch besides Magnesium Stearate. Drying record of starch was also examined. Capsule cells, after removal of the content, were examined for water content and data compared with that of the retention samples of empty capsules and drug product. The marked difference in water content was observed in the capsule cell and the content of capsules of the complaint sample!

Assignable Reason

The water content was analysed in the complaint samples and retention samples of i) 50 empty capsules, ii) an equal number of complaint samples – the content of capsules and iii) that in the empty capsules shells after removal of the content were examined. The data was compiled for comparison. The average water content in each of the above was worked out and compared.

The data revealed that an increase in weight of the content of capsules in complaint samples was comparable to that of the loss of weight in the corresponding empty capsule shells. The average weight of filled capsules was found same as reported in the original QC report, both in the complaint and retention samples.

It was evident from the investigations that water from the hard gelatine capsules shell was transmitted to the content of capsules, which tallied with loss of water in corresponding capsule shell and hence there was a corresponding increase in weight of the content of capsules of the complaint samples.

Further scrutiny of the transit data logger information revealed that the temperature inside the container had gone up to 50°C for ten days!

The matter was also investigated with the shipping company with regard to storage of the container for ten days before being loaded into the ship. It was indicated that there was an issue before the ship sailed and hence, the container remained in the open for ten days in Mumbai dock!

All the data were shared with the QP of the testing laboratory. He agreed with the investigation and the observations. QP suggested us to inform MCA (present MHRA). We took up the matter with MCA, informing them of the issue along with all the data of investigations carried out, followed by tripartite (QP, MCA and Organisation) telephonic discussion. Both QP and MCA agreed with our observation and conclusion. We requested both MCA and QP that since the batch complies with all specification of BP, QP may release the batch with details of complete investigations attached to the batch record. A copy of the report was also filed with the batch record in MCA file for the next inspection.

Both MCA and QP were requested and agreed, and the batch was released by the QP for distribution and sale. Both QP and MCA agreed and closed the complaint.

CAPA

i. Relevant SOPs were amended. Deviation form was filed with the batch record.

ii. Water content in dried starch was specified as a part of IPQC.

iii. Weight of content of capsules was added to stability studies data.

iv. Transporters were advised that any delay in despatch beyond five days be intimated to us.

v. Data logger range of transit temp and RH excursion was recorded in the BMR.

CASE Study 6

Cephalexin Capsules BP 500 mg.

The organisation was exporting the product to several counties for the last five years. The product was well-received by the international market. The product pack was also exported to the East Asian country over a period of three years and well-received.

Product pack profile

Fifteen Cephalexin Capsules BP 500 mg, were blister packed using 0.025 mm thick heat seal coated printed aluminium foil with 0.25 mm thick PVC. Twenty blister packs were packed in a corrugated box of 3ply, 150 GSM craft paper. The box was sealed with adhesive tape. One and a half million capsules of the drug product, along with data logger, were shipped to the East Asian country by sea.

The customer from the East Asian country reported complaint of the product packs – quite few blister packs had deformed capsules and blisters of the product!

The complainant was acknowledged on receipt, indicating that we will revert with the assignable reason and the investigation report in four to six weeks.

Investigation

The local representative of the organisation in the East Asian country was requested to provide information from the customer i) details of the product, ii) the batch no., iii) mfg. date, iv) expiry date, v) the total quantity of the batch received vi) number of defective product packs encountered in the supply vii) was the complaint encountered in the original supply? viii) was there any onward transhipment? If yes, the mode and duration of transhipment, ix) quantity of the product transported and the complaint quantity.

The customer and local representative of the organisation were requested to provide few blister packs of complaints for investigation.

While awaiting the complaint samples, BMR and BPR of the batch were examined along with the retention samples of the batch drug product. All the documents and retention samples were found satisfactory.

For further investigation, we had to await the complaint samples. Samples were received – it was unbelievable to see the magnitude of deformed blisters and capsules therein. The samples were analysed and found to have degraded by 40 % of the drug content with darkening of the content of capsules!

It required significant thinking and investigation as to how could it have happened in about five boxes (100 blisters) out of 5000 boxes supplied in the consignment!

Telephonic conversation with the customer and the company representative revealed that five boxes of the total supply were transported to another customer by road. Further probing revealed that the products in the original corrugated boxes were transported in a metal box on a bicycle!

It was imperative to create a complaint in the laboratory to arrive at an assignable reason. A small batch of 3000 capsules of the product was prepared by R&D for the study and analysed as per BP. The capsules were blister packed exactly as supplied to the customer followed by packing in identical corrugated box. Two boxes each of 15 capsules x 20 blisters (300 capsules) were kept in i) accelerated stability chamber, 40°C and 75% RH, ii) at room temperature storage 25°C and 60% RH, iii) retention sample room, iv) balanced three boxes were kept at room temp for transit trial to be conducted.

Assignable Reason

The security department at the gate of the factory was informed of the transit test and the purpose. To simulate the transit condition, it was decided to keep three boxes in a dickey of the car with the data logger in one of the boxes. Every day, the car was driven a 45 Km distance each way and brought back to the factory, keeping the shippers in the dickey for five days as a worst-case scenario. After five days of transit test, shippers were brought back to QC-QA laboratory for examination/ observation to check for any damage during the simulated condition. i) The data logger revealed that the temp had gone up to 70°C for three hours every day for five days! The atmospheric temperature was 45°C for four hours midday. ii) All the three boxes were opened and blister packs taken out.

The transit test could reproduce identical damage in the shape of capsules and of the blister packs (they were photographed as evidence). The content of the capsules was found dark, and when analysed, as per BP, it was found to have 60% degradation with darkening of the colour of the content of the capsules, besides deformation of the capsules and the blister packs of the drug product similar to the complaint samples! No darkening of content of capsules, deformation of capsules and blisters were observed after five days in samples kept at i) 40°C and 75% RH, ii) at room temperature storage, 25°C and 60% RH and iii) retention sample room. Analysis of the drug content, as per BP, was found satisfactory and complied with the limits of Pharmacopoeia.

The customers and the company representative were provided with the data and details of the transit test along with photographs of blisters and capsules after transit test. It revealed that the market complaint samples were exposed to sever temp condition, which damaged the product – capsules and blister packs. The regulatory agency of the country was provided with a detailed investigation report of the product along with photographs of product packs, pre and post transit test.

A copy of the total investigation report and photographs of the product after transit test were sent to the customer and regulatory agency and also filed in the batch record of the product and in the regulatory agency file.

The customer was requested to reject all the complaint packs and written assurance for the same was obtained.

For good business relation practice, we provided a replacement. The customer agreed to the investigations and communicated closer of the complaint.

CAPA

i. SOP on international transportation was amended.

ii. Storage and transhipment condition for onward transportation – Not more than 30°C was indicated on the product pack.

iii. The above information was also included in the patient information leaflet (PIL) of the product pack.

All supervisors in production, QC, QA and packaging development, were trained with the observation of the case.

Export of Biotech Products to USSR (Russian countries)

The organisation had excellent export business in East European countries, including erstwhile USSR. The company was supplying a number of pharmaceutical products to USSR, including Human Insulin Injectable. The organisation had a technical tie-up with the US-based multinational company. A number of USP generic products were manufactured and supplied over the years. Products, including Human Insulin Injectable, were well-accepted by the country.

PACK PROFILE

Human Insulin Injectable products were exported regularly in 40 IU /ml strength, in 10ml vials of i) Insulin Human Injection USP, ii) Human Insulin – Isophane Suspension and iii) 70:30 (70% Insulin Isophane Suspension + 30% Human Insulin Injection). These products are extremely temp sensitive. Temp control was rigorously observed during manufacturing, filling in the vial, cold storage of vials till taken up for labelling of vials (storage at 2 to 8°C). Final labelling and packing in cartons with temp sensitive sticker indicator was affixed just before despatch followed by final packing: 12 such cartons were shrink-wrapped, and two such shrink-wrapped packs were packed in a thermocol box with coolant bags to maintain temp in transit which in turn was packed in a 150 GSM 3ply corrugated box. Two such boxes were packed in an outer corrugated box of 150 GSM 5ply craft paper. Products require refrigerated condition for storage till usage.

Before finalising the packs for export, ten shippers' dummy loads with identical packs with water for injection (since the products were very expensive) were subjected to transit test, along with a data logger, within India and brought back. They were examined for temp fluctuation during the transit and condition of packs. Transit test was found satisfactory with no damage to packs with the satisfactory condition of temp and dummies.

A total of sixty thousand vials of the above mentioned three products were exported to USSR. It was agreed with the customer to export the consignment to a destination by Air to Moscow.

All products were supplied to the regulator to the location in the USSR as per their instruction.

The USSR regulator complained that the location received the consignment with a 25-day delay and that some of the corrugated boxes were broken and the products were frozen!

The regulator was acknowledged receipt of the complaint, indicating that we would revert with the assignable reason and the investigation report in four to eight weeks since it was a case of international transport.

Investigation and Assignable Reason

Inquiry with the transporter – Air India revealed that the consignment was delayed because of a strike by Air India workers. Hence, the consignment was sent via Frankfurt on way to Moscow, without consulting the exporter!

For more details, it was decided to visit the location in USSR were the products were sent.

On reaching the destination – the outskirts of Moscow – the location manager showed damaged product packs. Yes, the customer was right. Some of the outer, inner boxes and thermocol boxes were badly damaged, exposing some of the vials to the atmosphere. The location manager informed that the consignment was received through a truck from Frankfurt, without temp control; it had met with an accident on the way! Some of the boxes fell down from the truck and were torn and exposed to atmospheric condition, outside temp was minus 30°C! The vials that were exposed to the atmosphere were frozen. Details of the truck, transporter, driver and address in Frankfurt, with a copy of the transport documents, were obtained from the location depot manager.

On request, the location manager agreed to segregate damaged shippers from other shippers. Vials from damaged shippers were removed to verify that the vials were frozen and it was agreed to provide a replacement.

The customer was requested to open other shippers that were not damaged to examine the condition of products therein – not frozen and repacked. Detail record of quantity, name of each product, respective B.No. manufacturing and expiry dates were made and signed by the representative of the customer and the supplier. The customer was requested to segregate good vials (not frozen) and store at 2°C to 8°C for further action to be taken in future.

10% of the supply (about 6000 vials) were frozen and requested to segregate for future action.

Documents were prepared with the above details in the format signed by both the parties. The replacement of damaged vials to be provided by the organisation was agreed and indicated in the report.

The regulatory agency in Moscow was visited with a copy of the detailed report along with the concerned manager of the customer's depot; pending the inclusion of the investigation with the transporters – at Frankfurt and Air India in Mumbai – the regulatory agency was briefed with the complete details and the investigation's report till then. The regulatory agency asked the depot manager for a sampling of the frozen vials and that of the good vials for analysis at their end. The good vials, once found satisfactory on analysis, were accepted by the regulator; the frozen vials were rejected.

The Air India cargo office in Mumbai was visited to discuss the issue of the consignment booked (Airway Bill) for transport by Air India to Moscow, sent via

Frankfurt without informing the consignor who exported the consignment!

The Air India cargo handling manager informed that the consignment booked for Moscow remained with them for more than 15 days due to strike by Air India workers! Air India decided to transport the consignment to Frankfurt by Lufthansa for onward transport to Moscow. From Frankfurt, there was no flight to Moscow for five days; hence, Air India, at Frankfurt and Lufthansa, decided to transport the consignment by road! All these decisions were made by Air India in Frankfurt and Mumbai and Lufthansa in Frankfurt without consulting the consignor party in Mumbai! A series of lapses/ blunders were committed due to lake of knowledge/ bother to look at storage condition indicated on even outer corrugated boxes! The written report was prepared and signed by the concerned manager of Air India and the consigner organisation. It was the highest level of negligence by Air India!

Lufthansa in Frankfurt was approached to find first-hand information. Air India handed over the consignment to Lufthansa in Mumbai for Moscow without ascertaining when it would reach Moscow! Lufthansa did not bother to read the storage requirement indicated on the outer boxes! At Frankfurt, the cargo was kept for five days since there was no flight to Moscow. To avoid demurrage, Lufthansa decided to transport the consignment to a destination near Moscow by road in a truck!

It was total failure/negligence and careless attitude of both Air India and Lufthansa!

A detailed report was prepared duly signed by Air India, Lufthansa and the consignor. A copy of the report was sent to the regulatory agency in Moscow.

On receipt of replacements of frozen vials, on our request to the regulatory agency in Moscow, agreed to close the complaint.

Action Taken

Legal notices were issued to both Air India and Lufthansa, followed by court case for negligence in their services, leading to damage to the consignment. An insurance claim was lodged, making Air India and Lufthansa accountable, which became a long-drawn issue.

CAPA

i. SOPs on the transport of goods were amended with clear instruction "No change in transportation rout and mode is permitted" than one agreed in the bill of lading.

ii. All bills of lading must indicate the temp storage condition required during transportation.

iii. All boxes must have symbols indicating "Life-Saving Medicines strictly follow storage condition indicated".

iv. Supply chain, warehouse, purchase, distribution/despatch, QA, QC, production and packaging supervisors were trained with the above case study.

Case Study 8

Managing Disaster in Pharma

❖·······················❖

The manufacturing unit of the organisation located near Ahmedabad, India was scheduled to be inspected by the International Regulatory Agency. Suddenly, on 26th Jan. 2001 (the 52nd Republic Day of India), 08:46 AM an earthquake took place in Gujarat state in India 6.9 Richter scale for about two minutes, devastating number of cities in the Gujarat state. Several buildings collapsed, killing thousands of people. Aftershocks continued for quite some time on the day and thereafter. People were shaken up by the rude shock.

Investigation and Plan of Action

By 9:15 AM, reconciled from the situation, Sr. Vice President Operation (SVPO) rushed to the pharmaceutical manufacturing unit, located at about 37 Km from Ahmedabad, to personally see the magnitude of damage to the property caused due to the earthquake!

The security person at the gate of the factory indicated what he saw during the earthquake. He described an almost 40° swing of the boiler chimney! The emergency services engineer on duty was called by the security personnel for help to take stock of the situation. The security person was asked to open the warehouse since it had six high stacking of goods on sturdy metal racks. The goods kept on the fifth and sixth racks had dropped on the floor, breaking glass bottles, spilling the liquid.

The next concern was of utility. The electrician on duty was told to check the power supply from the mains of government supply. It was there.

Next was the boiler. The base of the chimney foundation was checked – nuts were checked and tightened – and found not affected. The boiler attendant climbed up through rack-ladder on the chimney to verify all the joints that were not disturbed.

Water supply – the bore well was next. The engineer was cautioned to just inch only the power supply to verify that pipes and bore well were intact and not damaged by the earthquake. With four times inching of the power supply, he verified that the bore well was working and allowed the water to be pumped at least 15 minutes.

Next was the diesel generator set. The foundation bolts were checked to ensure they were not affected. The power supply inched three to four times before the generator was put on running mode to verify that it was in working condition.

Having been satisfied with working of engineering services, next was contacting all Sr. Managers – Engineering, Production, QA, QC, Warehouse, Distribution and PA to Sr. V.P. operation – requesting them to report to the manufacturing unit in about two hours to work out post-disaster management.

Such a disaster was not anticipated, and hence, there was no SOP for guidance. On arrival of all the persons, they were briefed of on the spot observations made.

The first attempt was to work out SOP on Post-Disaster Management. Each one of them was requested to work out post-disaster plan details of their respective area and included them in the SOP. SOP was reviewed, modified and finalised as tentative SOP.

Architect and Engineer (A&E), who had designed the manufacturing facility, was called and informed of the earthquake. He was requested to visit the plant at the earliest since cracks were observed on the external surface of walls in the building. The external visit of the plant was taken along with the A&E, which revealed cracks in the outer surfaces. He informed his people to come to Ahmedabad with the necessary Polysulfide putty sealant materials along with their testing equipment.

They verified that all the cracks were on the surface only, and no deep damage was noticed by the civil engineers on testing. All cracks were sealed and painted after a couple of days to ensure they did not open.

SOP was further amended to include civil work and rectification of surface cracks/damage.

Teams consisting of one person, each from engineering, QA, QC, and production, were made for each one of the areas – machinery and equipment-wise. Area-wise formats were designed for documentation to verify and enter the details of equipment, machinery, electricity supply, civil work in the room, foundation, wherever applicable, with a cautious approach. Each team was instructed that any abnormality observed, it should be brought to the notice of the concerned departmental head and rectified. Each format was signed by each team member and submitted to the departmental head and QA for verification and signature. It was finally submitted to SVPO for a critical view.

Special care was taken while verifying each one of the HVAC systems. The external agency was called for a total HVAC system revalidation. The water system, including purification, hot water circulation system and its temp and pure steam generator, were revalidated and documented. Temp mapping was redone in the warehouse. Media fill was carried out in each aseptic area.

The international regulator spoke to Sr. V.P. Operation to check whether it was safe to travel to Ahmedabad (India) given the earthquake. They were advised by their embassy in India to postpone their visit. On hearing/reading and seeing the information in media, they preferred to postpone their visit by a month.

People working in the plant were allowed to enter the areas after it was certified by engineers as safe for people and cleared by the respective teams including QA to start clean-up work.

The above documentation covered a total of six box files – area/activity/machinery wise record.

After about a month, regulators visited for inspection. After an initial discussion about the earthquake, SOP on post-disaster management was shown and mentioned that this was not anticipated and hence, there was no SOP. This SOP was made on the day of disaster. SOP and documents, six box files, covered all the activities carried out and observations made by the respective team. Having gone through the post-disaster management and actions taken, the regulators were satisfied. They indicated that for them, this was the first instance to inspect the organisation after a massive disaster.

During the inspection, they verified the above documents in the respective area to satisfy themselves, besides routine inspection work.

After three days of inspection, they mentioned that the measures taken by the organisation after the disaster were satisfactory. The inspection went well with a few suggestions.

CAPA

It was the first time to encounter such a disaster and undertake actions to ensure compliance. Voluminous six box files documents were a ready reckoner for future guidance. It is very important to establish compliance commitment and credibility to regulators.

CASE Study 9

Cefazolin for Injection USP

The organisation was regularly supplying Unit Lyophilised Cefazolin for Injection, USP to number of countries for quite some time. The product was well-accepted by a number of countries. A complaint was received from a customer in Geneva, who had supplied the product to Moscow, USSR, indicating that the batch complies with all the tests as per USP; however, it failed to comply with Reconstituted Solution Test of USP (found hazy).

The complaint was acknowledged, and 25 vials of the product were requested from the batch. Further, the customer was informed that we would revert with the investigation report in four weeks.

Investigation and Assignable Reason

The matter was given to QA in the organisation for investigation. Retention samples of the batch were taken out along with BMR and BPR for investigation. No apparent abnormality was observed.

The matter was referred for investigation to a team to find out what could have contributed to the issue –

raw materials, primary packaging materials – vials, rubber stoppers or the lyophilisation process?

On receipt, complaint samples, retention samples of the batch and previous five batches were subjected to reconstituted solution test as per USP. All the batches passed the reconstituted solution test except complaint samples and retention samples of the same. In case of complaint batch, some vials complied and some did not! Variation in the result of the test, within the batch, was observed!

Each one of the components – API, vials (pre-siliconised used), rubber stoppers (siliconised in-house) – were reanalysed as per specification. No abnormality was observed.

To reproduce the complaint in the lab, the same procedure as used in the production batch was followed. Water for injection was filled in vials, semi stoppered with siliconised rubber stoppers followed by lyophilisation. Vials were subjected to reconstituted solution test as per USP; they were shaken vigorously and left for five minutes. WFI turned slightly hazy! Further repeat trials were conducted, where also haziness was observed! All operators and supervisors were questioned for the result.

The operator who had siliconised rubber stoppers was asked to demonstrate the process with empty vials and rubber stoppers. The test was repeated, which revealed haze in WFI! It was siliconisation process of rubber stoppers with coarse dispersion of silicon responsible for incomplete siliconisation of rubber stoppers!

CAPA

i. Well-defined SOP was prepared indicating viscosity of silicon.

ii. The exact quantity of silicone fluid and rubber stoppers by weight included. Equipment to be used for micronisation was specified.

iii. Change control was made and approved by QA.

iv. Additionally, the test for the siliconisation of the rubber stoppers was to be certified by QA in every batch record as in-process control test.

v. The lyophilised product was to be critically examined by QA and certified in BMR as a part of in-process control.

Fresh three batches of the product were supervised by QA to ensure compliance. The batches were subjected to complete stability studies and found satisfactory in totality.

The investigation report, in the format, along with all the observations, was sent to the customer and regulator. In about two weeks, it was accepted.

On receipt of replacement of the complaint batch, the regulator was asked to close the complaint and return the quarantined batch, which they did. The complaint was closed.

CASE Study 10

Fluoxetine Tablets BP

❖∙∙∙∙∙∙∙∙∙∙∙∙∙∙∙∙∙∙∙∙∙∙∙∙∙∙∙∙∙∙∙∙❖

(Consultancy Project – Product for Export – In-house Issue)

Fluoxetine Tablets BP, 20 mg, batch size 200,000 tablets, was routinely manufactured and exported to a number of countries. It was well-accepted by overseas customers. A batch was under manufacturing and granules were analysed and approved for compression. About 5000 tablets were compressed initially to carry out quality compliance test as per Pharmacopoeia. The batch complied with all the tests but for dissolution test even on repeat test!

Investigation and Assignable Reason

The dissolution test was repeated, but this time, it was observed that some tablets dissolved; however, some did not comply! Doubts were raised in the way the dissolution test was carried out. Samples from the initial run were drawn by a QA supervisor and performed the dissolution test. He encountered a similar result of dissolutions test carried out earlier!

The QA manager was requested to get about 500 tablets out of the initial run of the product. These tablets were handpicked and divided into about 2 X 50 tablets groups. Two separate groups were given to QA for dissolution test, ensuring there was no mix-up. The results obtained amazed everybody since one group completely passed the dissolution test, and another failed completely! It intrigued everybody! How were they identified and segregated? This was the question everyone involved in the investigation was asking.

The tablet compression machine area, where it was compressed, was visited and the operator was asked whether he had dedicated sets of punches and dies for the product? "Yes, we have," he said. He was then asked whether he used the same set? "Sir, we have two different sets of the same dia." He presented set **A**, which was used for the batch and five damaged upper punches that were replaced with another set **B** from the machine, duly cleaned, for investigation.

Upper punches of both **A** and **B** were checked with a finger and thumb. The production supervisor was asked to bring a tool drawing of both the sets. When the supervisor and engineer were asked what they checked in the drawing since they had signed, there was no answer! "Can you explain the drawings? Did you check 'R' indicated in the drawings?" they were asked. Their silence was an indication that they had no idea! "Do you have the radius of Curvature gauge?" It looked they heard it for the first time!

The drawings were explained, and they were told to buy the Radius of Curvature (RC) Gauge, set of two (range), manufactured by a Japanese multinational company – Mitutoyo. The RC Gauges were purchased.

Training of Supervisors

Production operators, supervisors, engineers, production manager, QA and QC supervisors were familiarised with the machine/tool drawings. **R** indicated in the drawing was explained and its importance in the tools (upper and lower punches). The radius of curvature **R** measured using a male set of the gauge in upper and lower punches (deep concave) of new sets of **A** and **B** (shallow concave) and compared with one indicated in the respective drawing. They were made to feel between a finger and a thumb to make them understand that it was perceptible. **R** of compressed tablets was examined using a female set of RC gauge.

Set **A**, with a deep concave shape, will impart a low compacting force on granules against set **B**, with a shallow concave shape, which will exert a higher compacting force in the given setting, in tablet compression due to difference in the concavity of the shape of punches revealed in RC.

A completely new set of upper and lower punches, after measuring the RC of set **A**, was fixed in the tableting machine. The initial run was carried out manually and adjusted to the IPQC requirements and then a trial run of about 3000 tablets was taken using the granules previously used. The tablets were analysed for IPQC test, including assay and dissolution. The trial run was found satisfactory in totality followed by regular production under the supervision of QA, which was found satisfactory after meeting all quality standards – hard way to learn the basics of pharmaceutical engineering (PE)!

Several university teachers training programmes were conducted to train teachers on the importance of PE, which they had not studied!

QA was entrusted with training all R&D persons, tablet manufacturing area operators, supervisors, managers, supervisors of QA, IPQC and engineers. The training records were updated with this PE training.

CAPA

i.   Training SOP was amended to include use of radius of Curvature gauge.

ii. SOP was amended to include use of a full set of punches and dies and part replacement of punches was not permitted. Change control was made for each set of tools and respective drawing was again certified by the supervisors of tablet compression and the engineer.

iii. Copy of the deviation report and incidence report were included in the BMR with change control and training records.

iv. Importance of pharmaceutical engineering training in understanding the physics of tablet making.

Prostaglandin Analogue – Ophthalmic Drops

＊••••••••••••••••••••••••••••••••••＊

(Product for Export to Regulated Market – In-house R&D Issue)

A multinational organisation entrusted R&D work to develop ophthalmic drops of a prostaglandin analogue for marketing in the US and EU. The product and pack profile details were provided with a timeline for the introduction of the product in the agreement.

Plan of Action

An action plan for the project was made assigning the project to two R&D persons with well-defined responsibility.

1. Procurement of API and excipients from DMF sources.

2. Identification of primary packaging materials and procurement from DMF source.

3. Coordination with universities having lab facilities for High Pressure Homogeniser (HPH) and Nano-Sizer (NS) for particle size measurement.

4. USP specification to be followed for the API, excipients and that for primary packaging materials including a cap for the container.

5. Record keeping with page numbered register was finalised.

6. Training of R&D persons – Prostaglandin analogue USP requirements, Nano Technology (NT), HPH, NS and any other requirement emerge while working with the project.

7. Periodic progress report, every 15 days, to be submitted to the customer.

8. Once the project progress satisfactorily, procuring NS and HPH to be considered.

API was sourced (in small quantity since it was very expensive) from the East Asian country manufacturer having DMF and likewise excipients. Packaging materials were procured from DMF source in India. The required agreements were made with DMF sources for initial and subsequent requirements once the product is taken up for production.

Specification for API, excipients and primary packing materials were established as per USP with additional tests as per the supplier's specification.

R&D work was initiated using the in-house facilities available, to begin with. Two different universities were approached as they had i) HPH and ii) NS facility. Product – the process was established to meet the NS requirement. Later on, these facilities were developed in-house procuring HPH and NS.

Issues and Investigation

Development batches were prepared, analysed and filled in DMF sourced plastic containers and kept for stability studies. It was observed that the drug content was found depleted without degradation – no additional peak(s) was observed in HPLC analysis! The external surface of the containers was found wet! Further investigation revealed that the liquid was transmitted through micro pores in the plastic container, allowing nano-drug particles (in solution) transmission from the container wall, resulting in the depletion of drug content, though there was no degradation. The containers were labelled with a transparent label to prevent any breathing and transmission of the drug.

Since the product was found satisfactory, an additional quantity of API was procured from the same source. API was approved and used for further development batches. In the initial new batch, on analysis, it was observed to have an additional peak in HPLC analysis. However, the drug content was satisfactory without reflecting degradation! The API was reanalysed, which did not reveal any additional peak! A fresh batch was prepared to reconfirm the additional peak in the product!

The matter was taken up with the API manufacturer, who did not agree to have made any change! To reconfirm the results, a trial batch was repeated with a similar result! The API manufacturer was informed. On asking whether any change was made in synthesis? API manufacturer did not reveal any change they had made! They were told that the matter would be taken up with the US FDA since they were a DMF holder.

This brought the API manufacturer to their senses and they agreed to investigate the matter at their end. After a week, the manufacturer of API reverted with regret that, yes, they had made a change in the manufacturing site-location! A second supply was from the initial batch of the drug manufactured from the new site! They were questioned if they informed the US FDA and obtained their approval for change of location. The response was no! How could they do this with DMF-approved materials and then maintain that the material was compliant to the DMF? The manufacturer was embarrassed about such malpractice and on further insistence, agreed to provide free replacement of the API! After the receipt of replacement, they were told that the earlier material stands rejected and would not be returned. The manufacturer apologised for guff-up (or deliberate attempts!) at their end.

CAPA

i. SOPs on procuring DMF source API and any excipient were amended to include no change is permitted of site/rout of synthesis/equipment for DMF/any material unless approved by the US FDA or any other respective international regulator.

ii. For a new source of material, the initial trial development batch should be prepared before clearing the supply for R&D work.

iii. For the same material supplied from a different site of the same manufacturer must be treated as new source material.

iv. SOP on stability study was amended to include stability study of any products should be carried out with final labelling material to be used for the product to be marketed.

v. SOP on training was amended to include training of personnel from purchase/supply chain, warehouse, QC, QA, R&D and manufacturing with the case study and record to be maintained.

CASE Study 12

Amoxicillin Capsules BP

❖ ·· ❖

The product (500 mg) was regularly exported to the UK and other countries. It was well-accepted by overseas customers. In one of the supplies, QP reported about 2% lower assay than reported assay in the COA, although within the limit of Pharmacopoeia.

Product pack profile: Ten capsules (hard gelatine) were blister packed using heat seal coated 0.025mm thick hard tempered aluminium foil and 0.25 mm thick PVC; ten such blisters were packed in a printed duplex board carton along with PIL (patient information leaflet), and 20 such cartons were packed in a three-ply corrugated box of 150 GSM craft paper. Product – two million capsules were exported through a container service by sea with a data logger.

QP was acknowledged receipt of the complaint and informed that we would revert in four weeks.

Investigation

On receipt of the complaint, QA started an investigation and referred the BMR and BPR to look for any inadequacy in manufacturing and packaging! COA mentioned assay 99.2% and QP found as indicated 97.0%.

The customer was requested to send the data logger along with 100 capsules each from the top, middle and bottom layers of the consignment received at their end for our investigation and analysis to assess whether it was an issue in a top layer only or throughout the consignment!

QA started an investigation with retention samples of the drug product. Analysis data of the drug product complied with what was reported to the customer.

On receipt of awaited samples from three different layers, from the customer (identified by shipper number), they were labelled as top, middle and bottom samples and analysed as per BP. Assay report indicated in top layer 97.2%, middle layer 98.6% and the lower layer, it was found 99.0%. The data logger indicated that the temp had gone up to 45°C for 15 days. Stability data of validation batch were examined. It revealed that at 40°C and 75% RH in 12 weeks, the drug content was 97.0%.

On investigation with the transporter – Seaport – it was indicated that container was in the open atmosphere for 15 days before it was loaded in the ship.

Data and a detailed investigation report were sent to QP and MHRA, followed by a telephonic talk. Yes, the excursion of temp had resulted in the depletion of drug content, which was essentially due to an increase in temp as indicated in the data logger. However, the depletion in drug content was within the BP specification and in line with the stability data.

Both MHRA and QP agreed and accepted our investigation report, and on our request, released the batch for distribution and marketing. MHRA suggested that a copy of this report be attached to the BMR and so they could see it during the next inspection.

QP and MHRA also agreed to close the complaint and release the batch for distribution.

CAPA

i. SOP on transportation for export was amended to keep a track with air and seaport for a number of days; the container/consignment remained in the dock/port before actual despatch.

ii. QA was advised to keep track of the level of drug content at accelerated temp condition after 6 and 12 weeks.

CASE Study 13

Diclofenac Sodium Injection

❖⋯⋯⋯⋯⋯⋯⋯⋯⋯⋯❖

Diclofenac Sodium Injection in 2ml amber colour ampoule was manufactured and exported to a number of countries for several years. A customer from the East European country was supplied 50,000, 2ml ampoules by air. The customer complained that the consignment failed to comply with the particulate matter!

The customer complaint was acknowledged, indicating that we would revert in four to six weeks with a request to provide 100 ampoules of complaint samples for our investigation.

The product pack profile: 2ml (25mg/ml) product was supplied in an amber glass ampoule. Twenty labelled ampoules were packed in a honeycomb corrugated box of 150 gsm three-ply craft paper with honeycombed partition; each box was labelled and tapped. Forty boxes were packed in a corrugated box of 5ply 150 gsm, craft paper. The box was sealed with a tap followed by polypropylene carry strap.

Investigation

QA initiated investigation while awaiting complaint samples from the customer. BMR and BPR were scrutinised to find out any discrepancy was there in manufacturing or packaging. Retention samples of the batch were examined for pH, assay, particulate matter, microscopic examination and sterility.

On receipt of the complaint samples from the customer, samples were analysed for pH, assay, particulate matter, microscopic examination and sterility.

Complaint samples passed in pH, assay and sterility but didn't for particulate matter! Microscopic examination revealed minute crystals! These crystals did not appear like that of the drug.

R&D was assigned to prepare a 5L batch using the same AR number materials, which were used in the complaint batch. Washed sterilised ampoules were examined for particulate matter, which passed. The batch was sterilised by filtration and filled aseptically, followed by accelerated stability study.

Monographs in Pharmacopoeia of each material were examined, and the chemistry of each was looked at. The product contained Benzyl Alcohol and Propylene Glycol beside the drug. The chemistry of Benzyl Alcohol revealed that it was prone to oxidative degradation to Benzaldehyde, which in turn oxidises to Benzoic Acid. The complaint samples were centrifuged, and sediment was tested and found positive for Benzoic Acid.

The customer was informed of the complete investigation and corrective actions taken. Replacement of the product was provided, and the rejected stock of the product was destroyed under the supervision of the company's representative. A copy of the investigation and corrective actions taken were submitted to the regulatory agency.

CAPA

i.   Specification of Benzyl Alcohol was amended that freshly distilled material should be stored in a tightly closed amber glass bottle at 2°C - 8°C.

ii. BMR was also amended to ensure freshly distilled Benzyl Alcohol stored, as indicated above, and was only used for the product.

iii. R&D, QC, QA, production supervisors were trained for the property of Benzyl Alcohol.

Customer and regulatory agency were requested and agreed to close the complaint.

CASE Study 14

Cleaning Agent – Microbial Contamination

❧ ···························· ❦

(In-house issue)

GMP requires cleaning operation before undertaking the next activity using the same instrument/equipment/machinery/area. Rightly so, you need to remove traces of previous product/material before undertaking next operation using the same equipment/machinery/area/atmosphere. It requires a validated cleaning process for visible, chemical and microbiological cleaning.

The cleaning process and material were validated. After cleaning a few SS vessels, which passed visibly and chemically clean criteria, in microbiological testing, it was questionable! Swabs were taken again and tested. It failed again! The sampling technique was questioned! The result was the same, even after sampling by an expert. It was a serious issue for investigation and cleaning had to be stopped.

Investigation

1. QA and QC initiated the investigation.

2. All equipment cleaned on the day were segregated for microbiological testing. The result was the same!

3. Purified water was tested, which was found satisfactory microbiologically.

4. Approved cleaning liquid from a sampled container was tested for microbiology and found contaminated!

5. Cleaning agent tested as per SOP. Physico-chemical testing was found satisfactory.

6. Direct sampling from the 20L container was taken for microbiological testing, which was found heavily contaminated!

7. Reputed multinational manufacturer/supplier was informed and called for discussion.

8. MNC representative indicated that this product is looked after by their consumer division and they get the product from a SSI manufacturing unit (with questionable GMP!).

9. The manufacturer was informed that it was their responsibility to provide material with COA, including microbiological testing and absence of pathogens. The cleaning agent was rejected and blacklisting the manufacturer.

10. Change over to another validated brand cleaning agent resolved the issue.

11. All previously cleaned equipment were segregated and cleaned again with another validated cleaning agent followed by sanitisation with 70% IPA followed by air drying. All equipment were resampled for microbial testing, including pathogen and once found microbiologically satisfactory; they qualified for use.

CAPA

i. SOP on cleaning agent was amended to include microbiological specification with an absence of pathogens. The deviation report was prepared.

ii. The manufacturer of cleaning agent failed in microbiology was removed from the approved list.

iii. QA supervisor was retrained for microbiological swab sampling from equipment.

iv. Specification of all cleaning and sanitising agents were relooked to ensure microbiological testing covers total microbial counts and absence of pathogens and communicated to suppliers.

v. Manufacturers of cleaning agents were informed that the QA team would audit their facility once again and if found satisfactory, then only it would be reapproved.

Should we expand microbiology course content in pharmacy curriculum in line with requirements of Pharmacopoeia?

Pre-approval Inspection — Dilemma of Supervisor and Manager

→⋯⋯⋯⋯⋯⋯⋯⋯⋯⋯⋯⋯⋯←

(Consultancy Project)

The organisation had submitted ANDA to the US FDA for a generic drug product. The regulatory agency informed the organisation of the visit of their inspector, who was visiting for a pre-approval inspection.

The inspector went to different areas in the warehouse – rejected material area, QC, manufacturing, quarantine product area besides packaging area, document storage area, etc.

While going around the different areas, the inspector carried the documents submitted by the organisation in support of the ANDA. The inspector was accompanied by a senior manager of the organisation to assist/clarify any query/doubt. He had inquired about several aspects and verified the information submitted with actual practice. He did raise queries to the supervisors and departmental head to satisfy with regard to knowledge of supervisors and managers.

To assess and verify processes in the manufacturing area, he was accompanied by the consultant who was helping the organisation to train the operators, supervisors and managers on various aspects of cGMP, GLP, GEP and GxP requirements and periodic audit for compliance.

The inspector opened the BMR, called the supervisor and asked whether the BMR was signed by him? He said yes, he had supervised the batch and signed. The inspector then asked him to show him how he operates the rapid mixer granulator (RMG) mentioned in the BMR. He asked if it was the same unit that was used for the granulation of the batch? The supervisor said that it was. Then the inspector asked him to go ahead and show him how he operates the unit?

The supervisor went up the stand on which the RMG was located. He struggled to start! The consultant was with him for support. He fumbled while demonstrating the working! In the meantime, the departmental head entered the area. Seeing the supervisor's hesitation, the inspector asked the departmental head if he signed the BMR? When the head replied that he did, he was asked to demonstrate the working of the RMG. The supervisor came down from the RMG stand, and the departmental head went up. He also struggled to operate it. It looked like both the supervisor and the departmental head had no idea how to operate the unit!

The consultant talked to the operator in their local language and asked whether he had made the batch and signed the BMR? He said that he did. The consultant then politely told the inspector that he was the operator and had manufactured the batch. The inspector told the operator to demonstrate the operation of RMG. He went up with the consultant. The operator looked confident except that he could not speak English and was apprehensive. He was encouraged to speak in the local language and was told that the consultant would translate it in English. This was explained to the inspector, who appreciated and agreed.

The operator explained starting of the unit until completion of the operation, including the use of the ampere metre as process control for dry mixing and wet mixing. He also explained that, at the end of the operation, once the amperage indicated in the BMR is reached, it is the end point of granulation and the granules are evacuated in an FBD bowl. The inspector was satisfied with the explanation and thanked the operator without asking any further questions.

From the above experience, a **few questions emerge**:

1. As a technically qualified person, should supervisors and managers learn the machine operation and nitty-gritty of the process?

2. Should they be encouraged to learn pharmaceutical engineering of the machine operation they supervise?

3. Should these be part of pharmacy education? Who can do it, and how can it be done and implemented?

It reminds me of a comment of the US FDA inspector, in one of the technical sessions, if graduation in pharmacy is a prerequisite, by law for a job in Pharma industry, whether academia has a role (in imparting knowledge of machine operation)!

CAPA

i. SOP on the training of technical persons amended to include understanding and operation of machinery used in the area being supervised.

ii. All supervisors must be exposed to manufacturing minimum of three batches of a product using machinery as a part of appreciation and understanding of pharmaceutical engineering.

iii. Training record should be updated with actual working.

iv. After the inspection, special training was identified for individuals and training organised.

v. Could the Pharmacy Council of India/Academia help in revising the course content of pharmaceutical engineering!

Compulsory Use of Bar Code for Drugs and Drug Products

(This case study is not based on the experience of the author. However, he believes that this information support unbiased information revealed and legislated by the US FDA.)

With the title of this case study emerge reaction – do we need this? Dispassionate thinking will respond that the safety of a patient has to be part of any medical treatment. Medical error, reported or not reported, has been a serious threat throughout the world to any health care system. The USA Report of the Institute of Medicine in 1999 revealed that between 44,000 and 98,000 Americans die annually due to medical mistakes (1). In many countries, they may not have data on this issue!

Considering that medical error has been a serious issue that needs the attention of all concerned to the health care and safety of patient and cost associated with it to the exchequer, (US Media reported that wrong administration of iv infusion to patients cost $ 20 million per year for 20 years to exchequer), US FDA ruled on April 4, 2004, and made it mandatory to provide a barcode on labels of medication and biological products by the year 2006 (2). It was predicted that this would prevent 500,000 adverse events and transfusion errors over 20 years, with cost savings of $ 93 billion (3)!

This is an avoidable human error by the health care personnel, obviating the need to read the label, which is assured by the barcode reader.

This system has been adopted by the world over for drugs and drug products, which prevent human error and support the safety of the patient.

References

1. Kohn LT, Corrigan JM, Donaldson MS, editors, "To err is human": building a safer health system. A report of the Committee on Quality of Health Care in America, Institute of Medicine. Washington, DC: National Academy Press; 2000.

2. Food and Drug Administration: FDA issues barcode regulation; fact sheet. Washington, DC: 2004.

3. Department of Veterans Affair. Computerized Patient Record System (CPRS) technical manual, GUI version. In: VISTA (Veteran Health Information System & Technology Architecture) Health System Design & Development Documentation Library. Washington, DC: Department of Veterans Affairs; September, 2003:1-342.

CASE Study 17

Water Purification System – Use of Reverse Osmosis (RO)

⇢ ⋯⋯⋯⋯⋯⋯⋯⋯⋯⋯⋯⋯⋯⋯⋯ ⇠

The purification of water is being used even before GMP came into being. The simplest method of mere filtration was used in the pre-GMP era. With GMP in place, water purification was considered important. With progressive stages to cGMP, it was recognised that water purification plays an important role even in stability studies. With the advent to accelerated stability studies, it became mandatory to assure that impurities present in water have to be removed to assure the quality of product till self-life.

The number of permutation and combination of systems are being used in countries depending on the source of water, purification system(s) being used by the government in their purification process used for water supply to the public. Obviously, this depends on the quality of raw water and its source. Raw water and its source play a significant role in the selection of water purification system required. Each individual source and the location of the organisation has to be considered, and there is no zero fit approach in the purification system. If the source of water is from bore well(s) and the municipal water supply, with seasonal variation in the supply of water from the soil, it requires a robust system of purification to take care of unpredictable types and level of impurities.

The ultimate objective of the purification system is to meet the standards of Pharmacopoeia before purified water is used for any pharmaceutical purpose.

Organisation – Pharmaceutical Company, facility was previously approved by international regulatory agencies, engaged in manufacturing solid dosage forms and liquid injectable, located in New Mumbai. The organisation was exporting its products to regulated markets were expecting international regulatory inspection.

The inspector arrived and was introduced by the QA manager to the consultant, whose help was availed by the organisation for all technical aspects, besides the technical training of all levels of supervisors. The QA manager started the presentation of different systems with flow sheet diagrams. He presented water systems that were used for manufacturing purified water. The purification system involved sand filtration, followed by demineralisation plant, degasser and polisher with final exposure to UV before collecting purified water in a SS tank. The purified water was maintained at 70°C and kept in circulation loop in a turbulent flow.

The inspector asked for clarification and enquired if they had RO in their purification process. The QA manager responded that they didn't since they meet the standards of Pharmacopoeia with the existing purification system. The inspector repeatedly emphasised that they should have RO. The manager had no answer and politely kept quiet.

The consultant intervened and clarified that the organisation received the municipal water supply. Mumbai has a catchment area to collect rainwater and has, on an average, 100" of rainfall in about four months every year. This rainwater is filtered chlorinated before it is supplied by the municipality to the city. This water has on an average calcium equivalent hardness of about 50 and total dissolved solids (TDS) value of around 150. This is easily managed with the demineralisation plant.

Unlike Mumbai city, other cities have much higher TDS value above 1000 to 5000 and very high calcium equivalent hardness of around 300 to 1700. In such cases, you do require RO.

The inspector agreed on the rationale for not having RO.

It is very important to politely clarify these issues with data to international inspectors with systems prevailing in part of the city to avoid any misunderstanding.

CAPA

i. SOP on presentation of water systems was amended to clarify why the system is used to avoid queries.

ii. Supervisors of engineering, QC, QA and production were trained to understand with the rationale of any system being used.

CASE Study 18

Data Integrity (DI)

❖ ··· ❖

(In-house)

The issue of data integrity (Di) has attracted the attention of regulatory agencies world over. It is important to understand that Di is a part of CGMP, and hence, it requires compliance. Management commitment is a must for CGMP and is expected to ensure that data compiled are accurate and reliable.

In the 1980s, the FDA identified falsified data submitted in support of ANDA. Sequel to this, the US FDA focused on a pre-approval inspection to evaluate raw laboratory data submitted for ANDA to assess the capability of the site.

The US FDA guidance for industry (December 2018) clearly defines *data integrity* as the completeness, consistency and accuracy of data. Di is critical throughout the CGMP data life cycle. It is expected that *metadata* – information required to understand data has to be part of the document else data by itself is meaningless. It is expected that the person responsible for the *audit trail* should be aware of the system and of detecting questionable data.[1]

Over the years, Di related warning letters issued by the US FDA have increased from 4 in 2008 to 56 in 2017. A total of 152 warning letters were issued from 2008 to 2017 to industries in 13 countries! The highest numbers of warning letters received by the top three countries during 2008-2017 were India – 48, China – 43 and USA – 28.[2]

International regulators (WHO, MHRA, US FDA, EMA and PIC/S) have observed that CGMP violation involving Di has significantly increased.[3]

An in-depth study revealed that it was a compulsive habit that compelled an individual to indulge in the issue of data integrity instead of corrective action. This habit was cultivated by an individual, depending on the environment in which one was brought up. The acceptance level of a school teacher has a significant role in inculcating/encouraging/discouraging the wrong habit. Sometimes, lethargic attitude compels an individual.

The acceptance level or lack of supervision of the teacher(s)/supervisor(s)/economic consideration or quick-fix approach of the higher-ups plays an important role in encouraging/discouraging data integrity and consequently developing the culture for the same. This transcends to all levels depending on acceptance by the supervisor/higher-up.

In one of the scientific gatherings, an international regulator commented on whether academic institutions have a role in this? The genesis of the issue will stop at the door of academic institutions. In the rat race of fighting against time for academic achievement/business, strict action at the first instance will help in stamping the Di virus, subject to the courage of teacher/supervisor/ higher-up in preventing a disgrace to the organisation by a warning letter. Can it be done? It depends on the culture you want to encourage and establish.

It has been observed that the work of repetitive nature, such as the calibration of a pH metre or other simple units, attract data integrity issues besides an area where an individual would not like to reveal mistakes in manufacturing, testing including different chromatographic studies. In BA/BE studies, the stakes are high with the displeasure of the clients! It depends on organisational culture linked to commercial consideration. In the case of CRO, data integrity is quite an issue – x-ray plates, cardiograms, investigational biochemical analysis and data of BA/BE studies to mention a few. Individuals evaluating such areas have to be vigilant for possible data integrity issues.

Academic institutions have an economic/awareness issue in selecting electronic analytical balances – having the least count of 10mg and used for weighing less than10mg materials!

Out of the number of instances encountered in industry, one such instance of data integrity is presented here.

Case Study:

An organisation was approved by the international regulatory agencies. As per the requirement, the calibration of balances was a daily exercise required to be complied with, and the record has to be maintained. In the warehouse, in-warding of materials area, 300Kg certified balance was placed to verify the weights of the materials received. SOP indicated the balance to be used for minimum and maximum weight, indicating the capacity of the balance. Daily and biweekly calibration requirements were indicated in the SOP.

On the day of inspection by the consultant, the calibration record of the balance was shown duly certified by the operator and the supervisor. The operator was asked to verify all calibration carried out by him on the day. He explained that as per SOP, he used standard weights of 10Kg, 50kg, 100Kg and 300 kg (was used for full calibration once in two weeks). Recorded data by the operator indicated that the balance was within the limit of error permitted. The operator was asked to verify the full calibration carried out by him. He had no issue in verifying 10Kg, 50Kg. However, in the case of 100Kg and 300Kg, he could not even lift the standard weights! He was asked if he did it himself or asked for someone's help. He replied that he did it himself! But how could he have done it when he couldn't lift the 100kg and 300kg weights now? The operator and the supervisor were embarrassed as it was recorded as done with figures!

CAPA

i. Operator and supervisor were counselled that SOP does not restrict taking help in lifting the standard weights of 100kg and 300kg. Hence, he should have taken help for this and did it rather than entering fictitious data.

ii. Calibration record over one month revealed fictitious data records, which nobody had noticed!

iii. SOP was amended to indicate that for calibration, help could be taken for lifting (higher) standard weights.

iv. All operators and supervisors were trained to provide actual data and not indulge in fictitious data, which would be a violation of CGMP as data integrity is a part of CGMP.

The only solution is training without reprimanding individuals to an extent possible, making them understand that indulgence in data integrity violates CGMP and has credibility issue for individual and the organisation. Bringing a change in culture is a task by itself; someone has to shoulder the responsibility.

References

1. Data Integrity and Compliance With Drug CGMP, Questions and Answers, Guidance for Industry, prepared by the Office OF Pharmaceutical Quality and the Office of the Compliance in the Center for Drug Evaluation and Research in cooperation with the Center for Biologics Evaluation and Research,

the Center for Veterinary Medicine, and the Office of Regulatory Affairs at the Food and Drug Administration, December 2018.

2. PHARMACEUTICAL ONLINE, Guest Column, July 14, 2017, An Analysis of 2017 FDA Warning Letters on Data Integrity, By Barbara Unger, Unger Consulting Inc.

3. PHARMACEUTICAL ONLINE, Guest Column, December 13, 2016, Comparing Recent Data Management / Integrity Guidance From MHRA, WHO, & PIC/ S, By Barbara Unger, Unger Consulting Inc.

CASE Study 19

Transfer of Technology

❖·····································❖

(Consultancy Project)

The organisation was approved by several international regulatory agencies – the US FDA, MHRA, WHO, TGA, ANVISA, etc. They were exporting generic drug products to many countries. One of the importing countries in the EU was interested in having an agreement for the transfer of technology of some of the products they were regularly importing. The agreement was reached between organisations and documented for transferring technology for 12 drug products of four different drug molecules in uncoated tablets dosage form for filing the products with their regulatory agency.

Based on the agreement, protocols were made for each molecule and drug products thereof. The business partner was provided with each protocol and the timelines for product development studies. The technical head from the EU organisation agreed with the protocols and schedules provided.

The total laboratory work was distributed to four different product development pharmacists and an equal number of chemists from the analytical development department. A list of machinery, tablet tooling and equipment, including analytical instruments to be used, were provided to the customer for their information/comments/suggestions. The customer approved the list. It was decided and communicated that all DMF materials would be used and analysed as per BP, for the development studies, subsequent scale-up and production batches.

Development batches were prepared with a step-up- step-down concept for a common blend of each of the molecules – tablet tooling and the average weight of tablets, strength-wise, differentiated products within the molecule. Likewise, blister packing of each product, strength-wise within the molecule, were differentiated to avoid any mix-up at all stages of manufacturing, analysis and packing (by different colour printed label, foil and carton). Detailed BMR and BPR were made accordingly. Batches were analysed and once found satisfactory, kept on accelerated and long term stability studies as per ICH guidelines.

After six months of satisfactory stability studies at accelerated and long term stability conditions, the customer was informed. All BMRs, BPRs, analysis reports and stability data were shared with the customer for comments and suggestions.

After about three months, the customer responded, indicating their interest to take it forward for the transfer of technology.

The consultant was assisting for this technology transfer project from the beginning. All material specification, analytical methods, BMRs, BPRs, analytical reports and stability studies data were scrutinised.

Presentations by product development pharmacists, analytical development chemists, senior supervisors from QC and QA were made in a management meeting. It was agreed that all approaches in developing technology, process and analysis were in the right direction. The final decision was left to the consultant to plan out further course of action.

Training and Development

Product Development Pharmacists (PDP) and Analytical Development Chemists (ADC) indicated that they were ready for the transfer of technology. It was deliberated that, considering the batch size of 5000 tablets tried out for each of the products, do we need to take scale-up batch studies? Both PDP and ADC were confident that they did not need to scale-up batch studies. On enquiring, it was revealed that for the development studies, laboratory equipment/machinery was used! It was indicated by the consultant you had made baby batches for these studies and you would not be able to reproduce quality requirements at a production level! Remember you'll have different equipment, machinery, for a scale-up operation besides people once you go for a commercial scale. Hence, it is desirable to have scale-up batches where you'd transfer technology to in-house people using all production machinery and equipment. The analysis would be carried out by a regular quality control chemist, and the QA would supervise the processes. It was a tough decision for the success of the project. Remember, you'll be transferring technology to a different country, which may or may not have identical machinery, analytical equipment and tablet tooling and will have to train people who may or may not know English!

It was decided to take a common blend for 100,000 tablets for each of the four molecules with separate BMR using production facilities. Each common blend would then be subdivided into the respective products and treated as separate batches – BMR and BPR. All common blends and respective batches made thereof were monitored by the consultant to facilitate the preparation of the final BMR, respective BPR and analytical reports. It was also ensured that the concerned PDP and production supervisor learned the use of the machinery. Likewise, all analytical and in-process controls were carried out by regular QC and QA persons.

Having done and encountered the number of queries from production and QA, which were not anticipated, they had to clarify and find the answer for each one of them was a learning experience/training for individuals.

All the batches were kept on stability studies as per ICH guidelines. Once three months of satisfactory stability studies were observed, the customer was informed of the same, indicating that the organisation was ready for transferring technology.

The technical head of the recipient organisation responded, indicating that they would be glad to receive the team for transfer of technology.

The consultant and management decided who and how many persons would visit for the transfer of technology. The consultant suggested that, to begin with, we should send a team of four senior persons, one each from product development, QA, analytical development and a production supervisor, besides a coordinator from production. Two persons out of the group would come back after 15 days and would be substituted by two persons from respective areas of activity. The management insisted that the consultant be part of the team. The consultant put forward his views that he was confident of the team and would be in touch with the group leader every day. Any person in the team could contact him at any time. He further indicated that we need to develop the second line in command for the organisation. In the event of any eventuality, he would visit to resolve the issue, if any, for a successful transfer of technology and organisational commitment.

The team left for the destination; for many, it was their first experience of travelling abroad. They were confident.

The coordinator of the team (CT) was in contact with the consultant on reaching the destination and every evening. Training the trainer was their first task. Having gone round the facility of the customer, the team appreciated the tough job through which they had gone through in the organisation in India.

Every evening, the team would meet to discuss the issues faced, resolved and documented. The CT would provide feedback of the day to the consultant. Even the technical head of the customer (THC) would discuss with the consultant in India every alternate day. She was appreciative of knowledge of the team. The product and strength-wise new BMR, BPR and analytical protocol and formats were made and approved by the local QA and THC.

After 15 days, two persons from India were sent as replacement of two persons who returned. New replacements were briefed and trained by the CT with the equipment, machinery and the process change/ modification required for products already made.

The two who returned were appreciative of the host's cooperation. They appreciated the tough training they had undergone in India before visiting the customer, which helped them in their work. There was a change in their perception and approach to work.

Detail discussion used to be there with THC and she was inquisitive of the rationale of processes and acceptance of the concept of step-up-step-down by international regulators. It was clarified that the concept was well-accepted and used by the organisation in India while submitting ANDAs to US FDA, which were approved by the FDA. It was indicated that while implementing, you could make minor changes to the quantity of excipients in the formula with rationale to suit your requirements with supportive data and a deviation report under SUPAC guidelines. Any major change has to be supported with validation.

The batches manufactured and approved were kept on accelerated and long term stability studies, as per ICH guidelines, were found satisfactory. The product and strength-wise new BMR, BPR and analytical protocol, formats and COA were made and approved by the local QA and THC.

It took another fortnight to complete the transfer of technology for all four drugs and respective drug products.

There was a daily detailed discussion on the various aspects of technology transfer between the technical teams of both sides, along with THC to their satisfaction. All the decisions taken were documented and signed by THC and CT.

THC expressed her satisfaction in the transfer of technology to the consultant and appreciated the way it was done. The written document, to this effect, was made and signed by the THC and CT.

She requested that the consultant visit them during the launch of products. The consultant reciprocated the invitation to the THC to visit India and be our guest.

This was considered the first big international transfer of technology achievement for the organisation.

CASE Study 20

Paracetamol Tablets BP

The organisation was manufacturing and exporting Paracetamol Tablets BP to different countries in blister and bulk packs to regulated markets in the UK, EU and Middle Eastern countries since it had been approved by respective regulatory agencies.

Product Profile

As per the requirement of a customer, one million tablets in blister packs of 0.02mm aluminium foil and 0.25 PVC, each of 15 tablets, were exported to the Middle East. Twenty blister packs were packed in a printed duplex board box. Twenty duplex board boxes were packed in a 3 ply 150 gsm corrugated box, which was cello taped. The consignment was exported by air.

The customer complained that the product complied with the BP specification. However, it failed in the description!

The complaint was acknowledged, indicating that we would revert with the investigation in four weeks. The customer was requested to provide two boxes (40 blister packs) of the product for our investigation.

Investigation and Assignable Reason

Awaiting complaint samples, the QA started the investigation, examining BMR, BPR, retention samples and analytical reports of all raw and primary packing materials. No abnormality was observed.

On receipt of complaint samples, the tablets were physically examined. Few tablets revealed small black particles. What contributed these? Retention samples of the product and all materials were examined besides tableting machine tools. Some of the retention samples of the batch revealed black particles. A microscopic examination of all materials was carried out. Talc, used as a lubricant in the product, revealed black particles under the microscope, similar to that observed on few tablets of the complaint and the product's retention samples!

Retention samples of purified talc were examined. Small quantity – 5 G of purified talc was added to 100 ml of purified water and stirred for a couple of minutes to ensure that the material wets and allowed to settle. The bottom of the beaker revealed few black particles.

The manufacturer/supplier of the purified talc was called and told of the issue. The test indicated above was shown, which revealed black particles. The manufacturer indicated that talc is of natural origin. The material is milled followed by sifting through #60, analysed and packed.

R&D was advised to take five kg of purified talc and sift it through #100 and show the magnitude of black particles collected. It revealed that the practice of sifting of purified talc through #60 was inadequate to remove black particles. The manufacturer/supplier was advised that we amend the specification of purified talc to include sifting of the material through #100; it should be devoid of black particles.

CAPA

i.   Specification of purified talc was amended to include sifting of the material through 100 #, and there should be no black particles. Change control was made.

ii. Sedimentation test of 5% W/V of purified talc in purified water was included in the method of testing to ensure that sediment was free of black particles.

iii. To exhaust the existing inventory of purified talc, it was decided to sift through #100 to avoid black particles in any other product. The deviation form was filled up.

Investigation and assignable reason reports were provided to the customer. They were satisfied with the findings and CAPA taken. The quarantined product available with them was verified by the company's representative and destroyed at their end. Replacement of rejected product was provided.

The customer was requested to close the complaint and they closed it.

CASE Study 21

Hematinic Tablets

(In-house issue of 1977)

The organisation had been manufacturing and marketing hematinic tablets product containing Ferrous Fumarate, Folic Acid, Ascorbic Acid and Vitamin B12 for about two years. The product was well-accepted in the market.

A batch of the product was under manufacturing. Suddenly, the production supervisor informed the R&D that they were facing problems with the breaking of punches! The pharmacist who had developed the product went to the production floor to examine the issue but could not resolve it. The supervisor from R&D went to the production floor and tried to identify the assignable reason but could not help. The issue was referred to a team of R&D pharmacists, supervisors from production and QA to investigate.

Investigation and Assignable Reason

1. Production was stopped.

2. The pharmacist from R&D was asked to take up a batch of 5,000 tablets and use the tableting machine

in the production area with slow speed. Compression pressure was increased to get tablets as per specification. To begin with, it worked; however, on running the machine for a while, the issue resurfaced!

3. Same granules were tried on the tableting machine in the R&D lab. The issue was there!

4. It was decided to relook at the issue in totality.

5. The tablet tooling manufacturer was called to look from metallurgy angle and radius of curvature of tablets, but it did not help.

6. Granules of each of the API materials were prepared separately, using the same AR number materials as used in the production batch, to identify the culprit material. Granules of each API were compressed into tablets. All materials behaved normally except Ascorbic Acid!

7. When looked into the supplier/manufacturer, it was found that the materials department had purchased the material through STC (State Trading Corporation, Government of India), which controlled import of drugs in India at that time since the material was in acute short supply in the country! All imports of pharmaceutical materials were routed through STC and supplied to pharmaceutical manufacturers in the country. It was cost-effective for STC to purchase materials from East Asian country.

8. The material was sampled again and analysed. It complied with the specification of Pharmacopoeia!

9. R&D batch was taken using Ascorbic Acid, produced by an Indian manufacturer, the material used in earlier production batches. There was no compressibility issue! On repeating a batch with STC material, the issue resurfaced with compressibility!

10. Mesh size of Ascorbic Acid of both earlier Indian and East Asian origin was measured. Indian material was found to be of 80# size, and the imported material was found to be of 40# size. Except for particle size, both materials passed the specification of Pharmacopoeia.

11. It was decided to mill Ascorbic Acid of STC and Indian origin to 100# size, and both were processed separately to granules followed by compression. The issue appeared to have been resolved since both the materials could be compressed into tablets with normal speed!

12. All active materials including Ascorbic Acid from STC were sifted through 100#, except Ferrous Fumarate, which was sifted through 60# size. The R&D batch of 10,000 tablets was taken. Granules could be compressed into tablets using normal speed and even after increasing speed of the tableting machine.

13. A production batch of 100,000 tablets was taken with the above changes. The QA supervised the batch with deviation, documented in the batch record along with a copy of the investigation report. Compression of the batch was successful.

Corrective Actions (CAPA did not exist)

i. Master formula cards and process instructions were amended with change control.

ii. All active materials to be milled through Fitz mill (Indian Cad mill/Gansmill), hammer forward with 0.3 # to provide 100# materials.

iii. All excipients were passed through 60# as security sifting before processing of a batch as a safety measure as being done earlier.

iv. What went wrong? Granules did not have compressibility (due to coarse particles size of Ascorbic Acid), and to achieve compression, for tablet formation, compacting force was increased in the tableting machine beyond the limit! It resulted in the breaking of punches.

v. Excellent guidelines were derived from the book, *Tablet Making*, by Arthur Little and K.A. Mitchell, published by the Northern Publishing Co. Ltd. 1963. The book provided information – the correlation between punch tip diameter, the radius of curvature of the punch of tablet tooling and maximum compacting force on punch tips recommended (covering physics of tablet making). The book is no more published.

vi. Understanding and the approval of tablet tooling were emphasised. All R&D pharmacists, supervisors from production, engineering, QC and QA were trained based on the above experience, emphasising the role of micromeritics (particle size) in compressibility of products.

vii. Impact of micromeritics (particle size) in the physics of tablet making – compression – was a hard way to learn.

CASE Study 22

Antibiotic Powder for Oral Suspension

❖ ·· ❖

Consultancy

The organisation was manufacturing and marketing Co-Amoxiclave Powder for Oral Suspension USP. The product was developed and marketed in India.

Market complaints received were acknowledged from customers of lump formation of free-flowing antibiotic powder in a glass bottle with a ROPP cap.

The investigation, Assignable Reason and Action

The matter required in-depth investigation. The QA was requested to bring some of the complaint samples along with retention samples of the product. The BMR and BPR of complaint batch numbers were looked into. After looking at complaint and retention samples along with BMR and BPR, the protocol was made for investigation.

1. Five complaint samples were analysed for assay, moisture content, pH and viscosity. Drugs content were found – 50 to 60% of the label claim. The pH

had shifted beyond limit; the moisture content was out of specification! Moisture ingress in the container resulted in the degradation of drugs, change in pH and lump formation in containers. It was decided to recall all the complaint batches. The QA was advised to recall and stop production of the product.

2. Specification of primary packing materials – amber glass bottle and ROPP cap – were examined and found inadequate for the critical product!

3. The HDP bottle manufacturer, along with manufacturer of Child Resistant (CR) Cap, was called. They were requested to bring the drawing for HDP bottle and CR cap. They were examined and firmed up. CR cap required Induction Heat Sealing (IHS) Machine, which was also purchased.

4. R&D was advised to look into the composition of the formulation, besides the in-process control (ipc). Water Activity (WA) measurement (USP) was included as ipc. The revised manufacturing process was worked out to contain low moisture in the excipient granules followed by final blending with antibiotics. A dehumidifier was used to control RH in the area to $\leq 25\%$, and temp 20°-25°C.

5. Twenty HDP bottles were filled with 20ml purified water and capped with a CR cap.

6. The height of the HDP bottle with CR cap was adjusted in the IHS machine to ensure perfect sealing of wad on the mouth of the bottle with

80-90% current transmission from IHS machine on the cap. Sealed bottles were subjected to a leak test to ensure perfect sealing.

7. Once satisfied, R&D batch of the product was filled in clean, dry HDP bottles at ≤ 25% RH and temp of 20°-25°C, followed by capping using the CR cap and HIS and subjected to a vacuum leak test.

8. The R&D batch was kept on stability as per ICH guidelines. Once the batch was found satisfactory after three months of stability studies at accelerated conditions, production batch equivalent to 25,000 bottles was taken and monitored for stability studies.

9. Once accelerated stability studies found satisfactory, the product was reintroduced in the market with success.

CAPA

i. The technical team was advised that they should not introduce any product under pressure since it creates a wrong impression of the organisation in the market.

ii. Packaging development SOP was amended to include approval of drawing of all primary containers and closures such as bottles, vials, rubber stoppers, ampoules, tubes, caps, etc., with change control.

iii. SOP was made for water activity (WA) to be carried out for all critical products by QA. It was introduced as in-process control. All master BMRs were amended to include WA for all other critical products. QA was advised to ensure that water activity is carried out for every blend of powders with change control.

iv. SOP on in-process controls was amended to include water activity for blend and leak test for filled and sealed bottles.

v. SOP on critical product processing area – temp and RH – was amended with change control.

vi. All supervisors of R&D, QA, QC, engineering and production were trained to handle critical products processing with temp and RH control.

It is desirable to study the chemistry of drug(s) and integrate chemistry, engineering, processing and requirements of Pharmacopoeia.

CASE Study 23

Role of Excipient – Compressibility of Drugs

$$\rightarrow\!\cdots\!\cdots\!\cdots\!\cdots\!\cdots\!\leftarrow$$

(In-house issue – 1976)

The organisation was manufacturing and marketing chewable Antacid Tablets for several years. The product was well-received by medical professions and patients because of its acid neutralising and buffering capacity.

Label Claim: Dried Aluminium Hydroxide Gel 250 mg, Magnesium Hydroxide 250 mg and Simethicone 30mg.

The batch was under manufacturing and suddenly encountered no compressibility of granules! Several efforts by the production supervisor and assistance of the QA supervisor did not help! The issue was referred to the R&D supervisor, who could not resolve it!

The investigation, Assignable Reason and Action

1. It was decided to refer the issue to supervisors of R&D, production and QA to investigate. Production batch was stopped and quarantined.

2. BMR of the batch was scrutinised, providing no clues!

3. Analysis reports of all active and inactive ingredients were scrutinised, and no deviations were found.

4. The R&D supervisor was advised to take R&D batch of 5,000 tablets in the lab. The result was identical to that of production batch – no compressibility!

5. R&D trials i) active materials granulated, dried and attempted to compression in the lab using R&D compression machine. It could be compressed. ii) Granules were lubricated using the lubricant used in the production batch. The blend was not compressible!

6. The analysis report of the lubricant – Magnesium Stearate was examined. It was found satisfactory yet created a serious compressibility issue!

7. The specification given in the Pharmacopoeia was examined, and the results were compared with limits given in the Pharmacopoeia. It was within the specification!

8. When examined critically, it was found that material specification had a test for the congealing temperature – not more than 54°C.

9. When looked into the chemistry and specification given in USP, which indicated that it may contain not less than 40% Magnesium Stearate and a combination of Magnesium Stearate and Magnesium Palmitate, which should not be less than 90%. No mansion of remaining 10% material?

10. Further in-depth study of chemistry and manufacturing process followed by the manufacturer of Magnesium Stearate revealed that Stearic Acid obtained after hydrolysis of fixed oil was used for manufacturing Magnesium Stearate.

11. Study of hydrolysis of fixed oil revealed that depending on fixed oil used; it may contain a mixture of stearic, palmitic and oleic acids!

12. TLC study indicated that it contained Stearic, Palmitic and Oleic Acid.

13. When Congealing temp was reanalysed, it was found to be 54°C. The higher concentration of Oleic Acid would provide a congealing temperature closure to 54°. Oleic Acid is an oily liquid and provides an oily coat on granules on lubrication, making it difficult to compress.

14. Magnesium Stearate used in earlier batches was examined and found to have a congealing temp of 60°C.

15. R&D batch of 5,000 tablets of the product was made in the lab and a portion lubricated with Magnesium Stearate having congealing temp of i) 60°C and ii) 54°. Both granules were compressed to tablets separately in the lab. i) Granules were compressible to tablets; however, ii) could not be compressed!

16. New production batch of the product was manufactured using Magnesium Stearate, having congealing temp of 60°C, and blended for five

minutes. It was found satisfactory. The issue was resolved.

17. An integrated approach of chemistry and pharmaceutics, physics of tablet making, compaction behaviour of materials and the role of lubricant misbehaviour were learned hard way.

Corrective Action

1. Specification of Magnesium Stearate was amended for congealing temp as 60°-65°C. The manufacturer of the material was informed of the same.

2. SOP on material specification and analysis were amended with change control.

3. The BMRs of all products involving the use of Magnesium Stearate were amended for blending time of final granules after addition of Magnesium Stearate to maximum of five minutes with change control followed by stability studies.

4. Magnesium Stearate having congealing temp of 54°C was rejected and returned to the manufacturer.

5. Quality of excipients should not be taken for granted. It needs in-depth knowledge of its Chemistry.

European Pharmacopoeia was first to introduce different monographs for Magnesium Stearate, clearly defining its composition of Stearate and Palmitate, deleting the ambiguity of Oleic Acid. Other Pharmacopoeia followed the same over a period of time.

CASE Study 24

Hematinic Liquid with Innovative Packaging and Issues

································

(In-house issue 1975)

The organisation had been manufacturing and marketing Liquid Hematinic Product for a couple of years. However, marketing was not happy with the market growth potential of the product.

The Marketing Director (MKTD) discussed with the R&D head, whether something could be done to stimulate the growth of the product! Several alternatives were discussed, such as an improvement in taste, a change of packaging, making the product and packaging attractive and how to get a kick out of the product, etc. The R&D head asked the MKTD why not rejuvenate product in totality?

The MKTD said the product positioning would be Hematinic Liquid for family. The label claim of iron salt and vitamins would remain the same with 10% alcohol. No change in the label claim. The flavour, mouth feel and primary packing – amber glass bottle – were left to the R&D to decide. They were to ensure that the product was palatable and acceptable by children and adults – male and female members of a family. MKTD wanted to promote the product as tonic for family. Having considered the basic requirements of marketing, R&D worked out the action plan.

Plan of Action and Action Taken

1. Reformulation of the product in line with the requirements of MKTD.

2. Packaging research was advised to call glass bottle manufacturers for discussion.

3. Flavour manufacturer of international repute was invited for flavour(s) to be finalised.

4. Since there was no change in the label claim, there was no need to make a change in product permission from local FDA.

5. The use of sugar-sorbitol base with terpene less orange flavour gave a boost to the lingering palatability of the product. The product was outright preferred by the taste panel of 25 members and also approved by all concerned through sample approval form (SAF). The product was kept on accelerated stability studies in type II amber glass bottle, which was found satisfactory. This was followed by a scale-up batch, which was also subjected to stability studies in type II amber glass bottle and found satisfactory.

6. On the bottle front, several manufacturers were called, but they regretted when they were told we would like

to have amber glass bottle similar to imported whisky bottle (sample bottle shown). They were also told that the bottle should have swing characteristic with a 28mm ROPP neck – a tough task for any glass bottle manufacturer.

7. Ultimately, two glass bottle manufacturers agreed and provided a drawing. One manufacturer also provided wooden mock-up as per the drawing. Several changes were suggested in the drawing and mock-up of the bottle. Ultimately, it was an obtuse angle in base of the bottom of the bottle, which provided an effective swing characteristic in wooden mock-up with a flat surface on either side of the bottle for pasting label.

8. Once the shape of the amber glass type II bottle was finalised, change control form and SAF were circulated by the R&D, along with wooden mock-up of the bottle for 400ml pack of the product. It was circulated for approval to the heads of QC, QA, engineering, production, including packaging, director of the factory; respective directors of marketing (product management group, distribution, MKTD), finance, purchase, medical, personnel and finally managing director (MD). Everybody accepted the innovative change, but the production-packaging manager and supervisor didn't recommend a swing bottle as it would result in the breakage of bottles on the liquid filling line beside difficulty in labelling. However, it was overruled by the MKTD and MD. After consulting the R&D head, they went ahead with innovative packaging first time in Pharma industry in India.

9. Packaging research worked out corrugated box, for 12 bottles (4X3 arrangement) each of 400ml, of 5ply 150 gsm virgin craft paper, with a partition of 5 ply 150 gsm craft paper having a flap with a central hole to accommodate the neck of the bottle to prevent rattling in transit.

10. The transit test was carried out with ten shippers load (120 bottles), filled with purified water, on 550 km route involving two manual loadings unloading each way. The consignment, when returned, was examined by the QA for damage/breakage, but none was observed. The transit trial report was shared with all divisions concerned. The secondary packaging design was approved for implementation.

11. Production of the first batch of the product with a swing bottle was taken up. As anticipated by production packaging, there was breakage of the neck of filled bottles. The R&D head and packaging research supervisor went to the shop floor to study and rectify the issue. To study the exact reason for breakage, the product filling was stopped. Few bottles were filled with purified water and capped on line with ROPP cap to assess an assignable reason for breakage. It was a jerk during the movement of bottles on a conveyor belt, underneath ROPP capping machine, striking the neck of the bottle with head of the capping machine, breaking the neck of the bottles. The engineer was called and instructed to fix a jig on line to prevent rattling of the bottle before capping. Once the jig was fixed, the issue

was resolved. Trial after fixing the jig, 100 bottles filled with water was tried without any breakage of the neck. The regular liquid filling was resumed and supervised by R&D packaging supervisor for three hours. Once found satisfactory, a report was prepared for resolving the issue satisfactorily and signed by the supervisors of production packaging, engineering and R&D packaging.

12. The product with new packaging was cleared by the QA for despatch to different depots in the country.

13. The product pack was launched by marketing. It was well-received in the market, boosting the sale in three months. The MKTD was very happy with the feedback and sales pick up.

14. The feedback received by the R&D packaging from different depots in the country was of satisfactory receipts of the consignment.

15. Three months after introduction of the product with the innovative pack, suddenly, breakage of bottles complaints were received from Delhi depot in a number of consignments sent without indicating details of breakage!

16. A surprise visit to the Delhi depot by R&D head, coinciding with the despatch of a truckload of the product, was organised to receive the truck in Delhi depot. The depot manager was surprised and enquired of the sudden visit of R&D head! He was informed that the purpose of the visit was to have the Technical Audit of the depot and understand and analyse in-

transit breakage encountered in new product pack reported by you and find a solution to resolve the same.

17. A truckload of the product arrived and was getting offloaded. Not a single corrugated box had any breakage! The depot manager was confronted to show all broken bottles. It was informed that breakage was observed from the neck! On asking for broken necks, he could not show even a single broken neck or bottle! He was told that unless you submit a broken neck with intact ROPP cap of bottles, the complaint is not acceptable and is fictitious!

18. Depot manager was on the back foot and surrendered, saying, "Sir, since the product is so good and the bottle is very attractive, we receive several requests from government officials for the product, and we have to oblige!" The report was made for fictitious breakage of bottles reported by the depot manager to oblige government officials. The report was signed by the depot manager and R&D head.

19. The R&D head went to report the matter to MKTD and MD of the organisation besides the Director of Factory.

20. Marketing exploited the product pack with its marketing strategy, calling it a product for swinging health – this further help to boost sale.

21. A 300 ml pack for a physician sample was introduced, and a 100ml mini empty bottle was used with a plastic twig of the flower with a slogan "NUTRIFIL FOR

SWINGING HEALTH" to medical professionals. Product sale zoomed up to swing.

This is nothing uncommon and similar instances are encountered with the success story of a product in the industry.

CASE Study 25

Cefadroxil for Oral Suspension USP

(Aggrieved Customer – 1997)

The organisation was manufacturing and marketing cephalosporin products in India and exporting to a regulated market – the US, UK and number of other countries. The product was marketed in India in an amber glass bottle with a ROPP cap. It was well-received in the market.

Customer – a retired Col army officer – wrote a letter to the managing director (MD), expressing his anguish. The letter was forwarded to the locational head of the factory to respond. On receipt of the letter, the customer was contacted on the phone to acknowledge his letter, which was forwarded by the MD.

The customer had expressed his experience in dealing with the company's representative in a chemist shop. Once the organisation grows, people in the field get egocentric and behave arrogantly. This is frequently observed in the field. They don't care for the customer, forgetting that they earned their livelihood because of them.

The customer was contacted on the phone when he mentioned that his doctor had prescribed the product for his granddaughter. He had purchased four bottles of the product for treatment from a chemist. The child vomits out the product with the first dose! He indicated that the product had turned dark and partial lumpy with a foul smell. When reported to the chemist, he, in turn, introduced the customer to the company's representative, who happened to visit the chemist for orders of other products. He had arrogantly refused to accept the complaint! This compelled the customer to write to the MD. After hearing the customer, he was requested to send all the four bottles to the factory for investigations and was assured that we would send a replacement of the same through courier. The customer was appreciative of our gesture, which was a part of customer service. On receipt of four bottles from the factory, he called up and profusely thanked and returned the complaint samples for investigations. He wrote a letter of appreciation to the MD, which in turn was sent to me.

With one good gesture, you win the customer's loyalty to the company. Complaint samples were analysed and found ROPP cap was loose, resulting in the ingress of moisture, turning the product into lump formation and partial degradation. Observations were shared with the customer with a request to close the complaint. The complaint was closed.

CAPA

i. SOP on Environmental requirements in production was amended with respect to temp and RH to $23 \pm 2^{\circ}C$ and RH $35 \pm 5\%$. With a deviation form.

ii. SOP on the capping machine was amended to include periodical checks to ensure proper capping.

iii. Operators and supervisors in production and packaging line were trained with the case study.

Tablet Compression Machine

The organisation was approved by international regulatory agencies and was exporting different solid dosage forms, drug products – tablets – to regulated markets like the US, UK, Australia, South Africa, etc., besides catering to the domestic market. They had battery of tablet compression machines to cater to the requirements. All the tableting machines – 16 stations to 71 stations – were separated by individual close cubicles with independent air handling systems.

Some of the machines were dedicated to certain products. During one of the inspection rounds, one 16 station compression machine was making an abnormal compression sound! The operator was called and asked why there were unusual sounds from the machine? He responded by saying it was an old machine. The engineer looking after the machine was then called and questioned. He also replied the same as the operator.

Both the operator and engineer were told to go to the cubical, run the machine for at least 15 minutes and get back and report. After 15 minutes, they returned, saying that it was the normal sound of the machine! Both were instructed to go in again, stop the machine and open the lubrication box provided on the back of the machine and report. Both were surprised and reported that there was no grease in the box! The operator was instructed to remove the product from the machine and clean it. The engineer was asked to fill grease and run the machine for at least 15 minutes without the product and report back. To their surprise, the abnormal sound disappeared!

After the lubrication compression machine was run for 15 minutes and the compressed tablets were collected separately, the QA was asked to carry out all IPQC tests to verify whether there was any change in the IPQC data! No significant change was noticed. However, lubrication did help in reducing the stress on compaction.

CAPA

i.   SOP on lubrication of machine was amended to include periodic lubrication of machine and recorded in the format.

ii. Supervisors from production, engineering, QA and operators were trained to understand noise from the machine and need for lubrication. This was also included in the initial training of recruits.

Chewing Gum Based Mouth Fresheners

Consultancy Project

The organisation was manufacturing and marketing mouth fresheners – chewing gum based products – successfully for many years. Suddenly, they received consumer complaints indicating that the product left a bitter taste in the mouth! Since it was a consumer product and they received a number of complaints from consumers, the organisation could not take a chance. This impacted sales of the product and they could not overlook the complaints. The product was rejected and returned by stockists and other consumer retail outlets. Both the QA and production supervisors tried to find an assignable reason but could not.

The consultant was appointed to resolve the issue that had impacted the business. He was appraised of the issue and its impact on sales.

Investigation and Action Taken

1. Formulae of different products marketed were studied. The composition of each was compared, and retention samples of different products were analysed.

2. Since the complaint was of organoleptic nature, a taste panel was established, and people were trained for conducting a scientific evaluation of organoleptic of the product.

3. Twenty people, who were non-smokers, non-tobacco and pan chewers, non-liquor drinkers, were selected to evaluate their taste buds by subjecting them to double-blind evaluation to ensure they perceive the samples of dilute syrup solution with different flavour tastes in a concentration of 0.1 to 0.5% – with salty, bitters, sweet, spicy taste and blend of all.

4. Those who could correctly identify 80% of samples were included in the final taste panel of ten persons. The gum base used (natural latex) was tasted to ensure it was not bitter.

5. Each one of the ingredients used in the product was also evaluated for taste in 10% sugar syrup to verify that there was no abnormal/bitter taste observed. Shortlisted materials were compared with the same materials from other AR number used earlier.

6. Mix fruit flavour manufactured by a multinational company was suspected as culprit, which imparted distinct bitter taste comparable with complaint sample!

7. Low concentration – 0.25% of the existing flavour in stock – was tasted in combination with each one of other ingredients in 10% sugar syrup to verify whether any other ingredient in the product was influencing bitter taste? Citric acid significantly increased bitter taste of the flavour!

8. A flavour manufacturer was contacted for help, and they sent their technical person formulator (TPF). He was appraised of the issue and tasted the flavour and compared it with a fresh sample of the flavour brought with him.

9. He admitted that the existing inventory of the flavour had a bitter taste.

10. The in-depth study revealed that an in-house inventory of flavour for more than three months was built up to meet production requirement and market demands of the product. TPF recommended that inventory of any flavour should not be kept beyond three to four weeks. He informed that these flavours are chemically aldehyde and ketone; hence, it should not be kept for a long period.

11. On request, TPF agreed to provide a fresh stock of flavour and took back the old stock. He also advised to keep the flavours in an air-conditioned area and suggested they keep an inventory of not more than four weeks with the assurance that they would promptly supply the flavour on receipt of order.

12. Chemistry wise, all aldehydes undergo oxidative decomposition followed by polymerisation. It is these

oxidised and polymerised components that impart a change in flavour note and bitter taste.

13. The issue was resolved and the product reintroduced in the market.

CAPA

i. Specification of all flavours was amended to include i) storage in the AC ($25°\pm2°C$) ii) inventory should not be more than four weeks.

ii. Based on the procedure used for the taste panel, SOP was prepared for a selection of taste panel members and conducting the evaluation.

iii. BMRs of all products were amended to include CAUTION that the dispensed flavours must be utilised within two days in production.

BA/BE Studies

The organisation was approved by international regulatory agencies such as the US FDA, MHRA, TGA, ANVISA, etc. The organisation had CRO, R&D and manufacturing facilities in the location.

The CRO used to carry out BA/BE studies, essentially for clients, in a well-equipped facility, besides that of a need-based domestic product of the organisation.

A CRO scientist (CROS) and R&D pharmacist (R&DP) approached the locational head for permission to carry out a BA/BE study of a product developed by in-house R&D. It was indicated that they planned to start the study from the next morning. They were asked to show the batch record of the R&D batch along with supportive QC and QA approval reports. It was indicated that R&D batch of the product, batch size of 5000 uncoated tablets, having three months satisfactory stability data as per ICH guidelines was to be taken up for BA/BE studies.

Prerequisite Queries for Undertaking BA/BE Studies:

1. Can you reproduce 5,000 tablets batch size on a commercial level production batch of 100,000 tablets using production machinery?

2. You will require a change in the composition of formulation to suit production machinery.

3. Do you think that a BA/BE study of 5,000 tablets R&D batch will hold good for a commercial batch of the product? Except it is for academic research/for new drug discovery.

4. The R&DP, who developed the product, was also questioned.

5. In defence, CROS said, "Sir, we have recruited volunteers for the study and ethics committee has already approved the study."

6. Did you inform the members of your ethics committee of the basic requirements for undertaking BA/BE studies? Since they may not be pharmacists or have a pharmaceutical background! The in-house technical group must approve the BA/BE proposal before taking it to the ethics committee.

7. Are you aware of the total cost to the organisation for one BA/BE studies?

8. The head of CRO was out of the country, and the proposal had his consent!

9. The head of the CRO was contacted on the phone to verify whether he had cleared the project? He had and

even indicated that the ethics committee had cleared the project. He was asked whether he informed the ethics committee of the technical requirements and rationale thereof, since all of them may not have a pharmaceutical background.

10. What is the cost to the company if bio studies do not hold good for a commercial batch? It costs the company about Rs. 2 to 3 million per study depending on the molecule and number of volunteers involved!

11. The CRO head said, "Sir, we have recruited volunteers for this study. Volunteers were provided dinner and regretted explaining that we couldn't take up the study due to certain reason and would call them back when we're ready."

12. For technical studies, everything has a cost, which must be kept in mind by the technical group.

CAPA – For Domestic Products

i. SOP on BA/BE study was amended to have a scientific and technical rationale for undertaking BA/BE studies of the in-house product. A minimum batch size of different dosage forms that can be manufactured using production facility was indicated.

ii. The batch size of a drug for BA/BE study should be decided by a technical team (TT) consisting of the heads of R&D, production, QA and CRO. Except for exploratory academic research project of a new drug/new drug delivery system.

iii. SOP on briefing members of the ethics committee for BA/BE studies amended to include scientific and technical rationale requirements for undertaking BA/BE for the domestic product or any other study that involves human volunteers or animals.

iv. For every in-house product, BA/BE study should have commercial consideration and approval of the finance department to establish techno-commercial consideration.

CASE Study 29

Disposal of Expired Animal Feed Product and Pesticide Containers

⟶.......................................⟵

(Issues reported in 1980, encountered by other organisations)

The organisation was manufacturing pharmaceutical products for animal health care. Periodically, retention samples of various products were examined and the expired ones were taken out for disposal.

A newly appointed QC chemist was assigned the disposal of expired retention samples of animal feed product. The product had primary packing in a printed polythene bag. Eight to ten printed polythene bags, each containing 400 G, of expired animal feed were taken to the ravine of a river for disposal. Considering that ravine and river will take care of the disposal of the product!

The disposed of product attracted stray animals in the ravine that ate the same, resulting in the death of some of them! The address printed on the polythene bags helped with the traceability of the organisation by the regulatory agency, pollution control board and the owners of the dead animals. The QA person of the organisation was summoned by the regulatory agency and pollution control board for careless disposal of the product. The organisation had to pay compensation to the owner of dead animals, and legal action was taken by the regulatory agency and pollution control board.

A **pesticide** manufacturing company had imported intermediates, for manufacturing pesticides, in metal drums of 250L capacity. Empty drums after use of intermediates were discarded for disposal.

These discarded drums were taken by nomads for storage. Some of the drums were used for storage of water and some for storage of grains. Stored water and grains were used for regular consumption for cooking! Traces of intermediates present in water and cooked food when consumed by people resulting in a poisonous effect on human systems, leading to adverse reactions and some deaths! This created regulatory actions by the government and pollution control board.

Lessons Learned from Others' Experience:

1. Disposal of expired goods should be undertaken by a trained, knowledgeable person only as per SOP.

2. Used containers of chemical intermediates should be destroyed and not to be sold as scrap.

3. In the chemical industry, ignorance is not bliss.

4. Due consideration must be given to impact on environmental/pollution control.

CASE Study 30

Rectification of Transferred Technology to Affiliate

············

A multinational organisation in India had transferred technology to one of its affiliates in Europe. The recipient organisation was not able to produce the product consistently. The aggrieved organisation requested the affiliate to rectify and resubmit the dossier.

One of the postgraduate students from the industry requested the author for help in refining the technology to resolve the issue and revising the dossier for resubmission to the affiliate.

The drug used was potent and small dose. The issue was studied in-depth, assuring confidentiality. It was noticed that the dossier was made in a hurry, overlooking the criticality of the drug and reproducibility. Rectification was undertaken without altering the formulation details.

Stepwise Rectification:

1. The development batch of 5,000 tablets was taken. All materials were sifted through #100 and the

materials, which could not pass through #100, were milled through Fitz mill, 0.3 mm mesh, with hammer forward.

2. The drug was mixed with an equal quantity of major excipient and sifted through #100.

3. The above-sifted material was mixed with an equal quantity of remaining quantity of excipient and again sifted through #100 and blended manually in a polythene bag.

4. The remaining quantity of previously sifted excipient through #100 was added to the blender containing the above blend and blended slowly.

5. A lubricant (sifted through #100) was added to the blend and blended for five minutes.

6. The blend was analysed for content uniformity by QC, which passed the test.

7. The blend was compressed into tablets on 16 station tableting machine at a medium speed.

8. In-process control tests, content uniformity, dissolution test and assay passed satisfactorily.

9. QC tested the final batch and found satisfactory in totality.

10. The next step was to repeat the batch with a batch size of 10,000 tablets with exactly identical process indicated above. The batch was found satisfactory.

11. The next two batches were taken with batch size each of 25,000 tablets to ensure repeat performance of the

process. Both the batches were found satisfactory in totality.

12. The next step was to embark on a regular batch size of 100,000 tablets. Once the batch complied with QC requirements, two repeat batches were made to validate the process to assure satisfactory process development and finalise the dossier.

13. The recipient organisation was requested to follow exactly the process and validate at their end. The revised dossier was well-accepted with excellent reproducibility.

CAPA

i. Separate SOP for potent/low dose drug processing was made, indicating criticality of process and importance of content uniformity.

ii. While manufacturing such product process, it should be ensured that the process does not create any segregation.

iii. The product process involves a dry operation and needs to be handled carefully with medium speed operation on the tablet compression machine.

Recommended Regulatory References

1. Drugs and Cosmetics Act 1940 and Rules 1945, Medical Devices Rules, 2017, By S W Deshpande and Nilesh Gandhi, Susmit Publishers, 9th Edition – 2018.

2. Government of India, Ministry of Health and Family Welfare (Department of Health), The Drugs and Cosmetics Act 1940 (As amended up to the 31st December, 2016) and The Drugs and Cosmetics Rules 1945 (As amended up to the 31st December, 2016).

3. US, 21 CFR Part 210—Current Good Manufacturing Practice In Manufacturing, Processing, Packing, or Holding of Drugs;

4. US, 21 CFR Part 211—Current Good Manufacturing Practice For Finished Pharmaceuticals.

5. Data Integrity and Compliance with Drug CGMP Questions and Answer Guidance for Industry, U.S. Department of Health and Human Services Food and Drug Administration, Center for Drug Evaluation and Research (CDER), Center for Biologics Evaluation

and Research (CBER) Center for Veterinary Medicine (CVM), December 2018, Pharmaceutical Quality/Manufacturing Standards (CGMP).

6. Rules and Guidance for Pharmaceutical Manufacturers and Distributors 2017, (Orange Guide) Medicines and Healthcare Products Regulatory Agency (MHRA), Published by Pharmaceutical Press, London.

7. EUROPEAN COMMISSION HEALTH AND FOOD SAFETY DIRECTORATE GENERAL, Volume 2A, CHAPTER 1 MARKETING AUTHORISATION, July 2019.

8. EudraLex – Volume 3 – Scientific guidelines for medicinal products For human use.

9. Annex 2, WHO good manufacturing practices for pharmaceutical products: main principles (Revision of WHO Good manufacturing practices for pharmaceutical products published in WHO Technical Report Series, No. 961, 2011, Annex 3).

10. Appendix 4: Disposal of unused / Expired pharmaceutical products, National Formulary of India, 2011, Indian Pharmacopoeia Commission, Government of India.

11. ICH Guidelines - Quality, Safety, Efficacy and Multidisciplinary (QSEM) Guidelines:

Q1A - Q1F Stability,

Q2 - Analytical Validation,

Q3A - Q3D Impurities

Q4 - Q4B Pharmacopoeias

Q5A - Q5E Quality of Biotechnological Products

Q6A - Q6B Specifications

Q7 - Good Manufacturing Practice

Q8 - Pharmaceutical Development

Q9 - Quality Risk Management

Q10 - Pharmaceutical Quality System

Q11 - Development and Manufacture of Drug Substances

Q12 - Lifecycle Management

Q13 - Continuous Manufacturing of Drug Substances and Drug Products

Q14 - Analytical Procedure Development

Integration of Regulatory in Pharma Sci.

The pharmaceutical industry is heavily regulated all over the world since the products manufactured are used for human beings and animals. Remember, there is nothing called seconds in pharmaceutical products. Regulatory science is a part of the pharmaceutical sciences, yet it is looked at in isolation. It needs to be linked with every subject in an academic institution to establish understanding by students that it has relevance in regulatory compliance. If you analyse global menace of data integrity, it reveals it has reached several countries in the world in its purview. For the industry, it is difficult to control since it is inherited from academia!

The question of whether we require integration of regulatory? Then emerges, how do we do it? Academicians will have to train students to establish linkage. Once it is done, students will understand its relevance. This is desirable considering the fact that students consider regulatory science as a necessary evil! This wrong notion has to be removed to facilitate working in the industry and other allied areas.

Regulatory compliance is a mandatory requirement for activities carried in pharmaceutical sciences by pharmacists in pharmacy, industry – warehousing, dispensing, manufacturing, packaging, analysis, bio studies, herbal products, health care products, neutraceuticals, dispensing of drugs at retail and wholesale outlets, hospitals, R&D, cosmetics and herbal drug cultivation including marketing and distribution. This is required to ensure accountability of pharmacist to regulatory compliance, including documentation.

Let us look, subject wise, at how we can interlink regulatory.

1. **Pharmaceutical Chemistry** – Be it synthesis or analysis, including documentation, it has to be in compliance with regulatory requirements **(Schedule M and Y) of Drugs and Cosmetics Act and Rules (D&CAR)**. Understanding Pharmacopoeial requirements as a legal requirement should be inculcated right from the beginning of pharmacy education. Academicians will have to have grass-root level **training and monitoring** to discourage ruthlessly issue of data integrity. Students, if left to them, will indulge in **data integrity** – manipulation! If this is left unattended, the wrong habits die hard and will be practised everywhere even while working even in the industry.

2. **Analytical Chemistry** – Precision working is a must and students tend to manipulate unless encouraged to be honest and not penalised them

for the wrong result. The habit of documentation (D&CAR) has to be insisted for the good of the profession, which covers the use of **sophisticated instruments** also. The use of **automated digital** systems tempts to manipulate incorrect results right in the system! This is a serious issue observed by international regulators, and they catch it by working on the system with trace back; remember, the regulator is experienced and takes no time to trace back level of manipulation. Close monitoring, creating awareness and correcting students to use individual pass ward are desirable. Reprimanding may not work. **Heavy metal analysis** to be linked with Pharmacopoeial (regulatory) requirements and is critical for the stability of drugs, products and adverse reaction in the body. This is neglected in **Ayurvedic/Herbal products** despite the inclusion in monographic requirements. Products are rejected on account of heavy metals by international regulators and destroyed (including food products).

3. **Pharmaceutics** – Dispensing requires a high level of precision and knowledge. An error in dispensing practical, I have heard the teacher saying that the patient is dead and you cannot avoid reprimand for the same. Here it is knowledge linked to regulatory requirements is desirable. In **technology,** the sequence of operation and processing involves the knowledge of **environmental control requirement** and familiarity with processing machinery and their

material of construction. This is linked with the compatibility/reactivity of drug(s) with contact metal parts with Pharmacopoeial standards applicable to the dosage forms. Present knowledge of **pharmaceutical engineering** imparted does not help unless radical change is brought in line with the requirements of the industry. This has limited the entry of pharmacists in Bio-medical, Medical Devices and Artificial Intelligence (AI) industries.

Poor understanding of the **process/pharma machinery** linked to regulatory knowledge is the culprit. Frequent reference to Pharmacopoeia can help in regulatory compliance. Regulatory is involved even in **package design**, stability studies and transit tests. Selection of packaging materials for every dosage form is linked with the property of packaging materials to meet the regulatory standard. **Microbiology** requirements, although critical, are neglected due to poor consideration in the course content. It is a part of regulatory requirements in total quality consideration. This has restricted the employability of pharmacists in fermentation, vaccine and biotechnology industries. **Environmental control and effluent treatment** requirements are regulatory compulsion.

4. **Pharmacognosy, Phytochemistry, Neutraceuticals and Herbal** – These are linked with the study of drugs of natural origin. Well-defined requirements are listed in Pharmacopoeia

with regulatory controls required. However, the **standardisation and compliance** for a repeat performance of therapeutic effectiveness have been an issue. The world has recognised these products, yet the level of quality confidence is questionable! The western world would like to shift to these products provided it assures **quality, safety and therapeutic efficacy with reproducibility of results.**

5. **Pharmacology, BA, BE and Clinical Studies** – These are the areas that have shaken up regulatory confidence due to issues of **data integrity** (manipulation) with questionable reliability of results. Lack of understanding in technical/ regulatory requirements beside dishonesty has created a serious doubt on the level of reliability of results. Should we aquent members of the **ethics** committee (who are not with a pharmaceutical background) with technical requirements of products before undertaking approval for **bio studies**? Academics have to find answer for these serious issues which have shaken up **confidence of regulatory agencies** at an international level. Can academia help rebuild the confidence of regulators?

The author has attempted some of the areas for the **integration of regulatory** with **different subjects in pharmaceutical sciences** to bring home the issue. It is a serious issue that needs the **attention of echelons of pharmaceutical sciences.**

www.ingramcontent.com/pod-product-compliance
Lightning Source LLC
Chambersburg PA
CBHW021415210526
45463CB00001B/374